SO-AWH-728

McGraw-Hill's

500 MCAT
Physics Questions
to Know by Test Day

Also in McGraw-Hill's 500 Questions Series

McGraw-Hill's 500 American Government Questions: Ace Your College Exams
McGraw-Hill's 500 College Algebra and Trigonometry Questions: Ace Your College Exams
McGraw-Hill's 500 College Biology Questions: Ace Your College Exams
McGraw-Hill's 500 College Calculus Questions: Ace Your College Exams
McGraw-Hill's 500 College Chemistry Questions: Ace Your College Exams
McGraw-Hill's 500 College Physics Questions: Ace Your College Exams
McGraw-Hill's 500 Differential Equations Questions: Ace Your College Exams
McGraw-Hill's 500 European History Questions: Ace Your College Exams
McGraw-Hill's 500 French Questions: Ace Your College Exams
McGraw-Hill's 500 Linear Algebra Questions: Ace Your College Exams
McGraw-Hill's 500 Macroeconomics Questions: Ace Your College Exams
McGraw-Hill's 500 Microeconomics Questions: Ace Your College Exams
McGraw-Hill's 500 Organic Chemistry Questions: Ace Your College Exams
McGraw-Hill's 500 Philosophy Questions: Ace Your College Exams
McGraw-Hill's 500 Physical Chemistry Questions: Ace Your College Exams
McGraw-Hill's 500 Precalculus Questions: Ace Your College Exams
McGraw-Hill's 500 Psychology Questions: Ace Your College Exams
McGraw-Hill's 500 Series 7 Exam Questions to Know by Test Day
McGraw-Hill's 500 Spanish Questions: Ace Your College Exams
McGraw-Hill's 500 U.S. History Questions, Volume 1: Ace Your College Exams
McGraw-Hill's 500 U.S. History Questions, Volume 2: Ace Your College Exams
McGraw-Hill's 500 World History Questions, Volume 1: Ace Your College Exams
McGraw-Hill's 500 World History Questions, Volume 2: Ace Your College Exams

McGraw-Hill's 500 MCAT Biology Questions to Know by Test Day
McGraw-Hill's 500 MCAT General Chemistry Questions to Know by Test Day
McGraw-Hill's 500 MCAT Organic Chemistry Questions to Know by Test Day

McGraw-Hill's

500 MCAT
Physics Questions
to Know by Test Day

Connie J. Wells

New York   Chicago   San Francisco   Athens   London   Madrid
Mexico City   Milan   New Delhi   Singapore   Sydney   Toronto

Connie Wells has taught physics for more than 20 years. She has served on the AP Physics Test Development Committee and, as a College Board institute consultant, has led workshops at teacher training institutes throughout the United States and abroad. She is chair of the Committee on Teacher Preparation for the American Association of Physics Teachers.

Copyright © 2013 by McGraw-Hill Education. All rights reserved. Printed in the United States of America. Except as permitted under the United States Copyright Act of 1976, no part of this publication may be reproduced or distributed in any form or by any means, or stored in a database or retrieval system, without the prior written permission of the publisher.

1 2 3 4 5 6 7 8 9 10 11 12 13 14 15 16 17   QFR/QFR   1 0 9 8 7 6 5 4 3

ISBN   978-0-07-179201-1
MHID   0-07-179201-5

e-ISBN   978-0-07-179202-8
e-MHID   0-07-179202-3

Library of Congress Control Number 2012938279

Illustrations by Cenveo

MCAT is a registered trademark of the Association of American Medical Colleges, which was not involved in the production of, and does not endorse, this product.

McGraw-Hill Education products are available at special quantity discounts to use as premiums and sales promotions or for use in corporate training programs. To contact a representative, please visit the Contact Us pages at www.mhprofessional.com.

This book is printed on acid-free paper.

CONTENTS

INTRODUCTION

Congratulations! You've taken a big step toward MCAT success by purchasing *McGraw-Hill's 500 MCAT Physics Questions to Know by Test Day*. We are here to help you take the next step and score high on your MCAT exam so you can get into the medical school of your choice!

This book gives you 500 MCAT-style multiple-choice questions that cover the most essential course material. Each question has a detailed answer explanation. These questions will give you valuable independent practice to supplement your regular textbook and the groundwork you have already covered in your physics class.

This book and the others in the series were written by expert teachers who know the MCAT inside and out and can identify crucial information as well as the kinds of questions that are most likely to appear on the exam.

You might be the kind of student who needs to study extra questions a few weeks before the exam for a final review. Or you might be the kind of student who puts off preparing until the last minute before the exam. No matter what your preparation style, you will surely benefit from reviewing these 500 questions, which closely parallel the content, format, and degree of difficulty of the questions on the actual MCAT exam. These questions and the explanations in the answer key are the ideal last-minute study tool for those final weeks before the test.

If you practice with all the questions and answers in this book, we are certain you will build the skills and confidence needed to excel on the MCAT. Good luck!

—Editors of McGraw-Hill Education

CHAPTER 1

Kinematics: Motion in One and Two Dimensions

Note: In this book, either $g = 9.8$ m/s² or $g = 10$ m/s² may be used in solutions that involve calculations. Since the answers are rounded, either value will provide the correct answer.

Dimensional and Graphical Analysis

1. Which of the following equations describing acceleration (a), displacement (s), time (t), and velocity (v) for a moving object could be dimensionally correct?

   (A) $a = \dfrac{vt^3}{s^2}$

   (B) $v = \dfrac{as}{t^2}$

   (C) $v^2 = as$

   (D) $t = \dfrac{v^2}{as}$

2. Which of the four graphs best represents a graph of "y as a function of x^2"?

   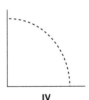

   I   II   III   IV

   (A) I
   (B) II
   (C) III
   (D) IV

3. On a graph that has a quantity measured in newtons on the *y* axis and a quantity measured in meters on the *x* axis, what units would identify the quantities associated with the slope and with the area?

   (A) The slope would have units of N/m and the area would have units of N·m.

   (B) The slope would have units of N·m and the area would have units of N/m.

   (C) The slope would have units of N and the area would have units of N·m.

   (D) The slope would have units of m/N and the area would have units of N·m.

4. Work is determined by multiplying force times distance. One joule of work is the equivalent of one newton of force multiplied by one meter. Which of the following is equivalent to one joule?

   (A) force = 5 N and distance = 200 cm

   (B) force = 5 N and distance = 20 cm

   (C) force = 50 N and distance = 0.2 cm

   (D) force = 5 N and distance = 2 cm

5. Quantities in everyday applications often have the prefixes *mega-* and *micro-*. How many micrometers (μm, sometimes called microns) are equivalent to one megameter (Mm)?

   (A) 1×10^3

   (B) 1×10^6

   (C) 1×10^{12}

   (D) 1×10^{15}

6. If quantity X is measured in kilograms, quantity Y is measured in meters per second, and quantity Z is measured in meters, determine the units on the calculated quantity.

$$\frac{XY^2}{Z}$$

   (A) $\dfrac{\text{kg} \cdot \text{m}}{\text{s}^2}$

   (B) $\dfrac{\text{kg} \cdot \text{m}^2}{\text{s}^2}$

   (C) $\dfrac{\text{kg} \cdot \text{m}}{\text{s}}$

   (D) $\dfrac{\text{kg} \cdot \text{m}^2}{\text{s}}$

7. If quantity X is measured in newtons and quantity Y is measured in kg/m, determine the units on the calculated quantity below.

$$\sqrt{\frac{X}{Y}}$$

(A) $\dfrac{\text{kg} \cdot \text{m}}{\text{s}}$

(B) $\sqrt{\dfrac{\text{kg} \cdot \text{m}}{\text{s}}}$

(C) $\sqrt{\dfrac{\text{kg} \cdot \text{m}^2}{\text{s}^2}}$

(D) $\dfrac{\text{m}}{\text{s}}$

8. The equation for the ideal gas law is $PV = nRT$, where P is pressure, V is volume, n is the number of moles of gas, R is the ideal gas constant, and T is temperature. Which of the four graphs best represents the plot of Pressure vs. Volume, where n, R, and T are constant?

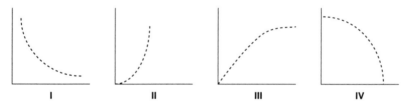

I   II   III   IV

(A) I
(B) II
(C) III
(D) IV

9. The equation for the period, T, of a pendulum with length L is

$$T = 2\pi \sqrt{\frac{L}{g}}$$

Which of the diagrams best represents data gathered for a pendulum with length as the independent variable and period as the dependent variable?

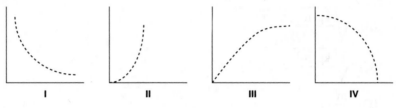

(A) I
(B) II
(C) III
(D) IV

10. Your professor provides you with data from an experiment. When you plot the data, it forms a curve of the shape shown here.

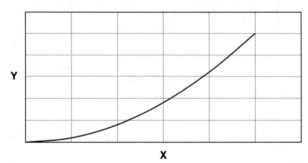

You are required to plot the data so that it forms a line (so that you can ultimately determine the slope of the line in order to find the equation of the line). How would you plot the data so that it forms a line?

(A) Y as a function of $1/X$
(B) Y as a function of X^2
(C) Y as a function of $\sqrt{X}$
(D) Y as a function of $1/X^2$

Vectors, Vector Components, and Vector Addition

11. What is the vector sum of vector X and vector Y?

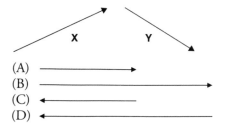

   (A)
   (B)
   (C)
   (D)

12. An airplane takes off at airport A, flies 300 km north, then 1,400 km at 45° north of east. After it lands at airport B, what is the closest approximation of the magnitude of the airplane's displacement from airport A?

   (A) 1,000 km north and 1,000 km east
   (B) 1,300 km north and 1,000 km east
   (C) 300 km north and 1,700 km east
   (D) 1,300 km north and 1,300 km east

13. Two perpendicular forces, a 30 N force directed due north and a 40 N force directed due east, are exerted simultaneously on an object whose mass is 35 kg. What is the magnitude of the resultant acceleration of the object in m/s²?

   (A) 155
   (B) 3.5
   (C) 1.4
   (D) 0.70

14. An airplane is flying north with an airspeed of 200 km/h when it meets a crosswind of 70 km/h toward the east. Which of the following expressions determines the resultant speed of the airplane?

   (A) $(200 + 70)$ km/h
   (B) $(200 - 70)$ km/h
   (C) $\sqrt{(200^2 + 70^2)}$ km/h
   (D) $\sqrt{(200^2 - 70^2)}$ km/h

15. What is the resultant of vector A minus vector B?

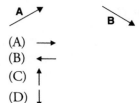

(A) →
(B) ←
(C) ↑
(D) ↓

Displacement, Velocity, and Acceleration

16. The graph illustrates the velocity of an object as a function of time.

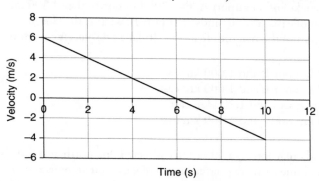

What is the object's instantaneous acceleration at $t = 5$ s?

(A) 0
(B) -2.5 m/s^2
(C) 1 m/s^2
(D) -1 m/s^2

17. An object starts from rest at $x = 0$ m and accelerates at a constant rate, moving from a position of $x = 0$ m to $x = 2$ m in 4 s. How far will the object move in the next four seconds?

(A) 3 m
(B) 4 m
(C) 5 m
(D) 6 m

18. The slope of a point on a Velocity as a Function of Time graph is

(A) change in position
(B) average acceleration
(C) instantaneous acceleration
(D) change in velocity

19. Which of the following could be true of an object moving with constant acceleration?
    (A) It moves in a circle.
    (B) It increases its velocity.
    (C) It decreases its velocity.
    (D) All of the above

20. A plot of Velocity as a Function of Time for a moving object is a straight line. Which of the following could be true?
    (A) The velocity is constant.
    (B) The acceleration is constant.
    (C) The acceleration and velocity are both zero.
    (D) All of the above

21. The path of an object's motion will be parabolic if it undergoes
    (A) constant velocity in two dimensions
    (B) constant acceleration in two dimensions
    (C) constant acceleration in one dimension and constant velocity in a second dimension
    (D) increasing acceleration in one dimension

22. Using the following graph of Velocity as a Function of Time for an object in motion, determine the change in position of the object over the first 6 seconds of its motion.

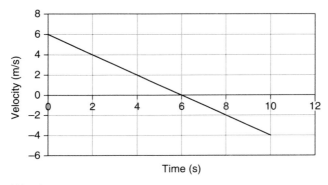

    (A) 0 m
    (B) 6 m
    (C) 18 m
    (D) 36 m

Refer to the graph for questions 23 and 24.

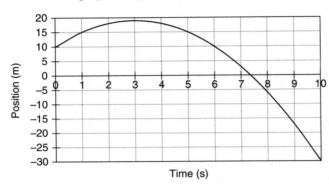

Time (s)

23. The graph describes the motion of an object as Position as a Function of Time. What is the best estimate of the velocity of the object at time $t = 7$ s?

    (A) 2 m/s
    (B) −2 m/s
    (C) 7 m/s
    (D) −7 m/s

24. In the graph, assume that the forward direction of the object is positive. What best describes the motion of the object?

    (A) The object moves forward for about 7 s, reverses direction at $t = 7$ s, and then moves backward for about 3 s.
    (B) The object moves forward for about 3 s, reverses direction at $t = 3$ s, and then moves backward for about 7 s.
    (C) The object speeds up for the first 3 s and then slows down during the period from $t = 3$ s to $t = 7$ s.
    (D) The object starts its motion by moving forward, then reverses its direction at $t = 3$ s and again at about $t = 7$ s.

Falling Objects

25. Which of the following best describes the acceleration and velocity vectors for an air rocket fired straight upward from the ground, from the moment just after it leaves the ground until it hits the ground again? Assume that the upward direction is positive.

    (A) The acceleration is always negative, and the velocity is positive on the way up and negative on the way down.
    (B) The acceleration and velocity vectors are both positive on the way up and both negative on the way down.
    (C) The acceleration and velocity vectors are both positive on the way up and on the way down.
    (D) The acceleration is always negative, and the velocity is always positive.

26. A ball is thrown into the air at a 60° angle to the ground, takes a parabolic path, and is in the air a total time of 4 s. If the upward direction from the ground is positive, what is the best estimate of the ball's velocity at a time 3 s after it leaves the ground?

    (A) +10 m/s
    (B) 0
    (C) −10 m/s
    (D) −15 m/s

27. A stone thrown straight upward has an acceleration that is

    (A) smaller than that of a stone thrown straight downward
    (B) the same as that of a stone thrown straight downward
    (C) greater than that of a stone thrown straight downward
    (D) zero until it reaches the highest point in its path

28. An airplane is flying horizontally at an altitude of 500 m when a wheel falls from it. If there were no air resistance, the wheel would strike the ground in

    (A) 10 s
    (B) 20 s
    (C) 50 s
    (D) 80 s

29. An air rocket is fired vertically at velocity v, rises to a height from the ground h, and remains in the air for a time t. When the same rocket is fired at v at an angle of 60° above the ground,

(A) the rocket reaches an altitude greater than h and is in the air for a time greater than t

(B) the rocket reaches an altitude less than h and is in the air for a time greater than t

(C) the rocket reaches an altitude less than h and is in the air for the same time as t

(D) the rocket reaches an altitude less than h and is in the air for a time less than t

30. A baseball is hit so that it rises almost vertically into the air. An observer counts a total time of 4 s from the time the ball is hit until it reaches the level of the baseball bat again. What is the best estimate of the velocity of the ball as it left the baseball bat?

(A) 10 m/s

(B) 20 m/s

(C) 30 m/s

(D) 40 m/s

Motion in Two Dimensions

31. A rock is thrown at velocity v horizontally from the top of a building of height h. How much time does it take the rock to travel from the edge of the building to the ground?

(A) $\sqrt{hv}$

(B) h/v

(C) $2h/g$

(D) $\sqrt{2h/g}$

32. The drawing shows the path of a projectile that is launched at an angle from the ground at point A and lands on the ground at point E. Assuming negligible air friction, at which points would you find an acceleration of zero, a maximum speed, and the maximum height?

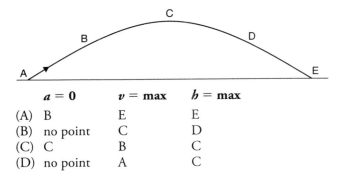

	$a = 0$	$v = $ **max**	$h = $ **max**
(A)	B	E	E
(B)	no point	C	D
(C)	C	B	C
(D)	no point	A	C

33. An airplane starts on a course due north at an airspeed of 100 km/h and encounters a crosswind from the west at 10 km/h. Which is the most likely resultant flight path of the airplane?

(A) 110 km/h on a path due northwest
(B) 110 km/h on a path due northeast
(C) 101 km/h on a path east of north
(D) 101 km/h on a path west of north

34. A boat that has a still-water speed of 8 m/s attempts to motor straight across a river that is flowing at a speed of 6 m/s. If the boat leaves the shore at point P, which of the vectors in the illustration represents the resultant path of the boat?

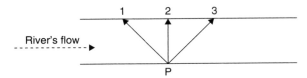

(A) path 1
(B) path 2
(C) path 3
(D) It is impossible for the boat to reach the other side of the river.

35. A block slides across a table and off the edge. What are the horizontal and vertical components of the block's acceleration from the time it leaves the table until it hits the floor?

(A) $a_H = 0$ and $a_V = 9.8$ m/s^2
(B) $a_H = 9.8$ m/s^2 and $a_V = 0$
(C) $a_H = 4.9$ m/s^2 and $a_V = 4.9$ m/s^2
(D) $a_H = 4.9$ m/s^2 and $a_V = 9.8$ m/s^2

36. A block slides across a flat roof that is 5 m from the ground and leaves the edge moving horizontally at a speed of 2 m/s. What are the horizontal and vertical components of the block's velocity when it hits the ground below?

(A) $v_H = 0$ and $v_V = 2$ m/s
(B) $v_H = 10$ m/s and $v_V = 10$ m/s
(C) $v_H = 2$ m/s and $v_V = 10$ m/s
(D) $v_H = 2$ m/s and $v_V = 14$ m/s

CHAPTER 2

Forces and Newton's Laws of Motion

Center of Mass

37. Three objects are shown on the grid, with the mass and coordinates of each object labeled. What are the coordinates of the center of mass of the system of the three objects?

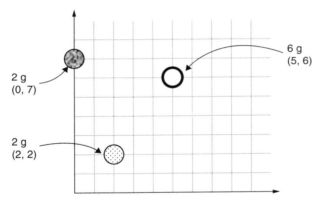

(A) 2.2, 4.0
(B) 3.4, 4.0
(C) 2.8, 5.0
(D) 3.4, 5.4

38. Three objects of equal mass are positioned on a coordinate plane at the *x*,*y* coordinates (2,6), (1,3), and (−6,−3). The center of mass on the plane for the system of three objects would be located at the point

(A) (0,0)
(B) (0,3)
(C) (3,0)
(D) (−1,2)

Newton's Laws of Motion

39. A 500 kg test car finishes a race and, because its brakes have failed completely, engages a parachute from the rear of the vehicle to slow down. Initially, it is traveling at 70 m/s, and in 4 s it has slowed down to 30 m/s. What is the magnitude of the average force exerted on the car by the parachute?

(A) 150 N
(B) 300 N
(C) 3,000 N
(D) 5,000 N

40. The graph plots data for the acceleration of an object as a function of the net force exerted on the object. What is the mass of the object?

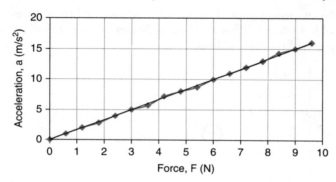

(A) 0.2 kg
(B) 0.6 kg
(C) 1.7 kg
(D) 2.4 kg

41. A truck towing a trailer accelerates on a level road. The amount of force that the truck exerts on the trailer is

(A) equal to the amount of force that the trailer exerts on the road
(B) greater than the amount of force that the trailer exerts on the truck
(C) equal to the amount of force that the trailer exerts on the truck
(D) equal to the amount of force that the road exerts on the trailer

42. A 2 kg cart is pulled across a horizontal surface. If the horizontal pulling force on the cart is 12 N when $a = 5$ m/s^2, what is the friction force of the surface on the cart?

(A) 0
(B) 0.5 N
(C) 1.0 N
(D) 2.0 N

43. A box is held stationary on a ramp by a string connected to the wall. The forces on the box are labeled in the diagram. Which of the following statements is true?

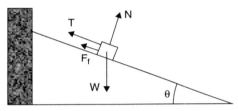

(A) $T = -F_f$
(B) $T = W \cos \theta + F_f$
(C) $W \sin \theta = T + F_f$
(D) $T + F_f = W$

44. A block is held by a string on a tilted ramp so that the block cannot slide. If the angle of the ramp is increased, how do the forces on the block change?

	Normal Force from Ramp	Static Friction	Tension from String
(A)	increases	increases	increases
(B)	decreases	decreases	decreases
(C)	increases	increases	decreases
(D)	decreases	decreases	increases

45. An elevator car weighing 10,000 N is supported by a steel cable. What is the tension in the cable when the elevator is being accelerated upward at a rate of 3 m/s^2?

(A) 13,000 N
(B) 10,000 N
(C) 7,000 N
(D) 4,000 N

46. An object with a mass of 15 kg has a net force of 10 N exerted on it. What will be the acceleration of the object in m/s²?

(A) 150
(B) 15
(C) 1.5
(D) 0.67

47. A net force of 10 N, applied for 5 s to an object with a mass of 2 kg, will change the speed of the object

(A) from rest to 12 m/s
(B) from 10 m/s to 25 m/s
(C) from 20 m/s to 50 m/s
(D) from 20 m/s to 45 m/s

48. Two perpendicular forces, one of 30 N directed due north and the second of 40 N directed due east, are exerted simultaneously on an object with a mass of 35 kg. Determine the magnitude of the resultant acceleration of the object (in m/s²) due to these forces.

(A) 155
(B) 3.5
(C) 2.1
(D) 1.4

49. A string of negligible mass connects three blocks on a level surface, as shown in the illustration. A force of 12 N is exerted on the system. Assuming no surface friction, what is the acceleration of the blocks and the tension in the string attached to the 1 kg block?

	Acceleration	Tension
(A)	4 m/s²	6 N
(B)	2 m/s²	2 N
(C)	2 m/s²	12 N
(D)	12 m/s²	6 N

50. A person is standing on a scale in an elevator car that is accelerating upward. Compare the reading on the scale to the person's actual weight (the gravitational force exerted by the Earth on the person).

   (A) The scale reading will always be the same as the person's weight.
   (B) The scale reading will be greater than the person's weight.
   (C) The scale reading will be less than the person's weight.
   (D) The scale will always read zero when the elevator is moving.

51. In the illustration, a picture frame suspended by two cords is at rest. Determine the value of the tension in cord 1.

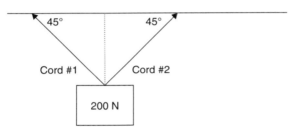

   (A) 50 N
   (B) 70 N
   (C) 140 N
   (D) 100 N

52. A force of 10 N is applied for 5 s to an object with a mass of 1 kg. The acceleration of the object is

   (A) 5 m/s²
   (B) 10 m/s²
   (C) 25 m/s²
   (D) 50 m/s²

Gravitational Force and Weight

53. A hypothetical planet has four times the mass of Earth but the same radius as Earth. If a rock weighs 12 N on the surface of Earth, how much would it weigh on the surface of the hypothetical planet?

   (A) 2 N
   (B) 6 N
   (C) 48 N
   (D) 12 N

54. A hypothetical planet has a mass half that of Earth (which has the gravitational acceleration g at the surface) and a radius twice that of Earth. What is g on the hypothetical planet?

   (A) $2g$
   (B) $g/8$
   (C) $g/2$
   (D) $g/4$

55. At a distance of 12,800 km from Earth's center, the acceleration due to gravity is about 2.5 m/s². What is the closest estimate of the acceleration due to gravity at a point 25,000 km from Earth's center?

   (A) 10.0 m/s²
   (B) 0.6 m/s²
   (C) 2.5 m/s²
   (D) 1.2 m/s²

56. Earth has a radius R. A satellite with a mass of 100 kg is inserted into an orbit at a position $4R$ above Earth's surface. What is the approximate "weight" of the satellite at this position?

   (A) $1,000$ N
   (B) 500 N
   (C) 400 N
   (D) 40 N

Spring Forces and Hooke's Law

57. A spring is compressed a distance of 0.10 m from its rest position and held in place while a 0.10 kg ball is placed at its end. When the spring is released, the ball leaves the spring traveling at 10 m/s. What is the spring constant?

   (A) 10 N/m
   (B) 50 N/m
   (C) 100 N/m
   (D) $1,000$ N/m

58. If a mass oscillating on a spring is halfway between its amplitude position and its equilibrium position, what percentage of its total mechanical energy is in the form of potential energy?

   (A) 0%
   (B) 25%
   (C) 50%
   (D) 100%

59. How much energy is stored in a spring ($k = 200$ N/m) when it is compressed by an external force 0.05 m from its rest position?

(A) 6.0 J

(B) 0.25 J

(C) 0.375 J

(D) 15.0 J

Static and Kinetic Friction

60. A string of negligible mass connects three blocks on a level surface, as shown in the illustration. A force of 12 N is exerted on the 3 kg block, and the friction force on each block is 1 N. What is the acceleration of the system of blocks and the tension in the string attached to the 1 kg block?

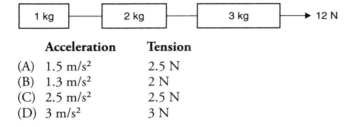

	Acceleration	**Tension**
(A)	1.5 m/s²	2.5 N
(B)	1.3 m/s²	2 N
(C)	2.5 m/s²	2.5 N
(D)	3 m/s²	3 N

61. In the illustration, a 20 kg box sits on a level table and is connected by a string to a hanging box with a mass of 10 kg. The coefficient of kinetic friction between the 20 kg mass and the table is 0.2. Assuming that the pulley has negligible mass and is essentially frictionless as it rotates, what is the tension in the string connecting the two boxes after the boxes start to move?

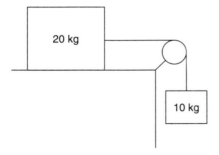

(A) 80 N

(B) 60 N

(C) 20 N

(D) 5 N

62. Which of the following statements is true regarding the coefficient of friction between an object and a level surface?

(A) The coefficient of friction is generally less than 1 if the object is moving and more than 1 if the object is stationary.

(B) As the object moves across the surface, the coefficient of friction decreases as the object slows down.

(C) The coefficient of friction is generally less if the object rolls than if the object slides across the surface.

(D) The coefficient of static friction is generally less than the coefficient of kinetic friction.

63. A 100 N box is pulled across a level floor with a constant horizontal force of 30 N, so that it accelerates uniformly at 2 m/s². Determine the friction force exerted by the floor on the box.

(A) 5 N

(B) 10 N

(C) 15 N

(D) 30 N

64. A box is sitting stationary on a ramp tilted at an angle of 30° to horizontal, which is the maximum angle at which the ramp can be tilted without the box sliding. The ramp is then tilted to a larger angle so that the box begins to slide. As the angle of the ramp is increased from 31° to 90°, what happens to the kinetic friction force and the normal force of the ramp on the box?

(A) The friction force decreases and the normal force decreases.

(B) The friction force increases and the normal force increases.

(C) The friction force remains constant and the normal force decreases.

(D) The friction force remains constant and the normal force remains constant.

65. Three boxes connected by strings, as shown in the illustration, are pulled across a level surface so that they accelerate at 0.5 m/s². The boxes are all made of the same material, so the coefficient of kinetic friction between each box and the surface is 0.1. What is the pulling force that is applied to the right of the 3 kg box?

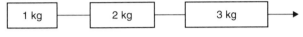

(A) 3 N
(B) 6 N
(C) 9 N
(D) 12 N

66. When a falling parachutist reaches terminal velocity, she is no longer accelerating. Which of the following statements is true about the parachutist?

(A) The gravitational force on the parachutist is equal to the friction force of the air on the parachutist.

(B) The gravitational force on the parachutist is still greater than the friction force of the air, so that the parachutist continues to fall.

(C) The friction force of the air on the parachutist has become greater than the gravitational force on the parachutist, so the parachutist no longer accelerates.

(D) The friction force of the air on the parachutist has reached a point where it no longer has an effect, so the parachutist falls at constant speed.

67. A force of 40 N is needed to set a 10 kg steel box moving across a wooden floor. Determine the coefficient of static friction between the box and the floor.

(A) 0.08
(B) 0.25
(C) 0.40
(D) 0.80

68. The force diagram defines the forces on a box sliding at constant speed down an inclined surface. Which of the following correctly expresses the coefficient of kinetic friction between the two surfaces?

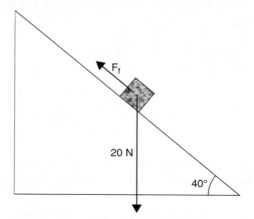

(A)   20 sin 40°

(B)   20 cos 40°

(C) $\dfrac{20 \sin 40°}{20 \cos 40°}$

(D) $\dfrac{20 \cos 40°}{20 \sin 40°}$

Mechanical Advantage and Pulley Systems

69. A lever is set up to lift a heavy box, as in the illustration. The box is set on one end of a board, and a large rock is placed under the board to act as a fulcrum. A force is applied downward at the opposite end of the board to lift the box. The box is at a distance l from the rock, and the force is applied at a distance of $3l$ from the rock. When the box is lifted a distance d at a speed v, what are the distance and speed for the force at the other end?

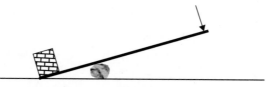

(A)   The distance is d and the speed is v.
(B)   The distance is $3d$ and the speed is v.
(C)   The distance is $3d$ and the speed is $3v$.
(D)   The distance is d and the speed is $3v$.

70. The illustration shows a pulley system with a fixed pulley attached at the top and a movable pulley at the bottom to which an object with weight W is attached. A rope is attached to the top pulley, wound around the bottom pulley, and then up and around the top pulley. Pulling down on the rope in the direction shown with a force F causes the object to be lifted upward. Assume constant speed, and neglect the masses of the pulleys and rope. When the force F moves downward a distance d, how far upward does the object move?

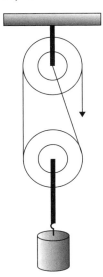

(A) d
(B) ½d
(C) ¼d
(D) 2d

71. The illustration shows a pulley system designed to lift an object of mass *m*. The system consists of a fixed pulley attached to the ceiling and a movable pulley to which the object is attached. What is the force that a person has to exert downward on the rope in order to lift the object at constant speed?

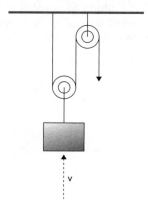

(A) *mg*
(B) ½*mg*
(C) ¼*mg*
(D) 2*mg*

72. A father and his two children play a game in which the children sit in a tire swing attached to a single rope that goes over a pulley attached to a tree limb, as in the illustration. The father stands on the ground, pulls down on one end of the rope and lifts the children sitting in the swing. The children, with a total mass of 40 kg, sit in the swing. With what force does the father pull downward on the rope to lift the children at constant speed?

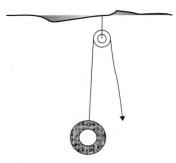

(A) 20 N
(B) 40 N
(C) 400 N
(D) 200 N

CHAPTER 3

Gravitation and Circular Motion

Gravitational Field

73. The gravitational acceleration g on the surface of a planet varies

  (A) in direct proportion to the planet's mass and in inverse proportion to its radius squared
  (B) in direct proportion to the planet's radius and in inverse proportion to its mass
  (C) in direct proportion to the square root of the planet's mass and in inverse proportion to the square root of its radius.
  (D) in direct proportion to the square root of the planet's radius and in inverse proportion to the square root of its mass

74. The weight of an object on the surface of Earth is 40 N. The radius of Earth is approximately 6,400 km. What would be the weight of the object if it were located 6,400 km above Earth's surface?

  (A) 40 N
  (B) 20 N
  (C) 10 N
  (D) 5 N

75. An object with a mass of 60 kg on the surface of Earth is taken to the moon, where the gravitational field value g is ⅙ that on Earth. What is the mass of the object on the surface of the moon?

  (A) 60 kg
  (B) 40 kg
  (C) 30 kg
  (D) 10 kg

76. The theoretical value of g on Earth's surface at the equator, based on the gravitational force between Earth and any object on its surface, is considered to be 9.8 m/s². However, the effective value of g is always slightly less, primarily due to

    (A) the effects of the sun and moon on our weight
    (B) the spin of Earth on its axis
    (C) a lack of knowledge about the exact mass of Earth
    (D) a lack of knowledge about the exact radius of Earth

Law of Gravitation

77. Two planets have the same density, but the radius of one of the planets is three times greater than that of the other. An object weighs 30 N on the surface of the smaller planet. What does it weigh on the surface of the larger planet?

    (A) 30 N
    (B) 60 N
    (C) 90 N
    (D) 270 N

78. Assume that the sun's mass is about 300,000 times the mass of Earth and that its radius is about 100 times Earth's radius. Compare the gravitational force on an object near the sun's surface to the gravitational force on the same object near Earth's surface.

    (A) 10,000 times
    (B) 3,000 times
    (C) 300 times
    (D) 30 times

79. Two objects have the same radius, but object B has twice the density of object A. A third object, C, is placed the same distance from object A as from object B. Compare the gravitational forces of objects A and B on object C.

    (A) Object B exerts twice the gravitational force on C.
    (B) Object B exerts half the gravitational force on C.
    (C) Objects A and B exert the same gravitational force on C.
    (D) Object B exerts four times the gravitational force on C.

80. Three objects are positioned along a line. Each has a mass of 2 kg and an x coordinate as shown in the illustration. Which object has the greatest net gravitational force on it due to the other two objects?

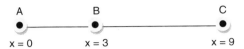

(A) The net force on A is the greatest.
(B) The net force on B is the greatest, and the net force on A is the same as the net force on C.
(C) The net force on C is the greatest.
(D) The net force on A is the same as the net force on C, and that net force is greater than the net force on B.

81. Three objects are positioned along a line. Each has a mass and x coordinate as shown in the illustration. Where could object B be positioned on the line so that no net gravitational force is exerted on it due to the other two objects?

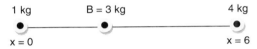

(A) at $x = 2$
(B) somewhere between $x = 2$ and $x = 4$
(C) at $x = 4$
(D) somewhere between $x = 4$ and $x = 6$

82. A satellite is in a circular orbit around Earth at an altitude of three Earth radii above the surface. Compare the gravitational force of Earth on the satellite at this altitude to the gravitational force of Earth on the satellite when it is sitting on the surface prior to launch.

(A) There is no gravitational force on the satellite when it is moving in orbit.
(B) The gravitational force is one half as great in orbit as on the surface of Earth.
(C) The gravitational force is one quarter as great in orbit as on the surface of Earth.
(D) The gravitational force is one sixteenth as great in orbit as on the surface of Earth.

83. Binary stars A and B have masses of m and $2m$, respectively. Compare the magnitude of the gravitational force the smaller star exerts on the larger star to the gravitational force the larger star exerts on the smaller star.

    (A) 1:1

    (B) 1:2

    (C) 2:1

    (D) 4:1

Uniform Circular Motion

84. When a satellite is in uniform circular orbit around Earth, what are the forces that must be exerted on the satellite to keep it in orbit?

    (A) None; the satellite needs no forces exerted on it to remain in orbit.

    (B) only the gravitational force of Earth on the satellite

    (C) the gravitational force of Earth on the satellite and a horizontal force to keep it moving

    (D) the gravitational force of Earth on the satellite and a centripetal force

85. A satellite is in circular orbit around Earth at an altitude of three Earth radii above the surface. If the satellite uses onboard retro rockets to cut its speed to one half, at what distance from Earth can it establish a new stable circular orbit?

    (A) between two Earth radii and three Earth radii above the surface

    (B) between three Earth radii and four Earth radii above the surface

    (C) less than two Earth radii above the surface

    (D) more than four Earth radii above the surface

86. An object is whirled in a vertical circular path by an attached string. For the speed of the object to remain constant at every point, the tension in the string must be

    (A) kept constant

    (B) greater when the object is at the top of its path

    (C) greater when the object is at the bottom of its path

    (D) zero at the top of its path

87. As an automobile turns a corner on a level road, the centripetal force necessary to keep the automobile in the turn is provided by
    (A) the gravitational force of Earth
    (B) the normal force of the road
    (C) the friction force of the road
    (D) inertia

88. A ball is whirled in a vertical circular path at a constant speed of 1 m/s. When the ball is at the bottom of the path, the string is cut. The ball will subsequently
    (A) drop vertically to the floor and hit the floor at a speed greater than 1 m/s
    (B) drop vertically to the floor and hit the floor at a speed less than 1 m/s
    (C) take a parabolic path to the floor and hit the floor at 1 m/s
    (D) take a parabolic path to the floor and hit the floor at a speed greater than 1 m/s

89. Student A is given a ball of mass m attached to a string of length R and told to whirl the ball on the string in a vertical circle so that its velocity at the top is at a minimum. Student B is given a ball of mass $2m$ attached to a string of length $2R$ and told to whirl the ball so that its speed matches the minimum speed of the one held by student A at the top of each ball's motion. In order to do this, student B must make sure that the string tension is
    (A) twice the tension as the one held by Student A
    (B) the same as the one held by Student A
    (C) half the tension as the one held by Student A
    (D) It's not possible under these conditions to match the velocities.

90. A nickel is placed on a turntable at a distance 10 cm from the center. When the turntable is set on 60 revolutions per minute, the nickel makes one revolution per second. What is the speed at which the nickel is moving in the circular path?
    (A) $2\pi/3$ m/s
    (B) 0.2π m/s
    (C) $\pi/2$ m/s
    (D) 0.1π m/s

91. A satellite with a mass m is moving at velocity v in a stable circular orbit around Earth, whose radius is R and whose mass is M. Which of the following expressions can be used to determine the satellite's altitude h above Earth's surface?

(A) $\dfrac{GM}{R+h} = v^2$

(B) $\dfrac{GM}{R+h} = v$

(C) $\dfrac{GM}{(R+h)^2} = v^2$

(D) $\dfrac{GM}{hR^2} = v^2$

92. Studies of traffic accidents on a particular curve lead to measures to reduce the number of vehicles going off the curve when the road is slick. Which of the following measures would be most effective in reducing such accidents?

(A) Reducing the speed limit for large vehicles, allowing only small vehicles to travel at regular speed.
(B) Creating a banked curve so that it slopes downward on the outside of the curve.
(C) Decreasing the radius of the curve so that the distance around the curve is less.
(D) Creating a banked curve so that it is higher on the outside of the curve.

93. As Earth rotates, the speed of a location on its equator is approximately 1,000 miles per hour. At what latitude would a location have half that speed?

(A) 30°
(B) 60°
(C) 45°
(D) 75°

94. A metal washer is placed on a turntable so that it just stays in place when the turntable is spinning. At this position, the washer is 10 cm from the center and is moving at constant speed. When the washer is positioned farther from the center, it slides off when the turntable is turned on. If the turntable always moves at the same speed, what must be done to allow the washer to stay in place when it is moved to 12 cm from the center?

(A) Glue another washer on top of the first washer.
(B) Sand the top of the washer so that it has the same surface on the bottom but has less mass.
(C) Scratch the bottom of the washer so that it has a rougher surface but same mass.
(D) There are no changes that can be made under these conditions that would allow the washer to move in a stable circle at a distance greater than 10 cm.

95. As a simple pendulum (an object that has mass and is attached to the end of a string) swings in a circular arc at an amplitude less than 90°, the tension in the string must

(A) remain constant
(B) be greatest when the object is at the bottom of its swing
(C) be least when the object is at the bottom of its swing
(D) be zero when the object reaches its maximum amplitude during the swing

96. Which of the following is NOT true regarding a satellite in circular orbit at constant speed around a planet?

(A) The centripetal force on the satellite is always toward the center of the planet.
(B) The satellite exerts the same amount of force on the planet as the planet exerts on the satellite.
(C) The force that the satellite exerts on the planet is in the same ratio to the force that the planet exerts on the satellite as the ratio of their masses.
(D) The acceleration of the satellite as it moves in its orbit is not zero.

97. In the diagram, a hollow cone is spinning horizontally on its tip and a small object inside the cone takes a circular path without sliding down the interior of the cone. Which of the following statements is a reasonable explanation for this situation?

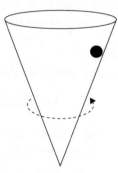

(A) The normal force of the cone on the object has a component toward the center that provides a centripetal force.

(B) The friction force of the cone on the object has a component that provides a centripetal force.

(C) The weight of the object has a component that provides a centripetal force.

(D) The combination of friction and the gravitational force on the object keeps it moving in a circle.

98. An object at the end of a string is whirled in a horizontal circle at constant speed, as in the diagram. If the mass of the object is 250 grams and the angle θ is equal to $60°$, which of the following expressions allows you to solve for the tension (T) in the string in newtons?

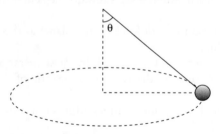

(A) $T = 0.25 \text{ g}$

(B) $T = \dfrac{0.25 \text{ g}}{\sin 60°}$

(C) $T = \dfrac{0.25 \text{ g}}{\cos 60°}$

(D) $T = 0.25 \text{ g} \, (\tan 60°)$

99. The moon's mass is about one sixth that of Earth. Compared to the gravitational force that Earth exerts on the moon, the gravitational force that the moon exerts on Earth is

   (A) one sixth as much
   (B) one half as much
   (C) the same
   (D) twice as much

100. A space shuttle in circular orbit needs to shift to a new orbit in which the astronauts experience a lower value of *g*. To accomplish this, the shuttle will stabilize in a new orbit

   (A) closer to Earth and at a higher speed
   (B) farther from Earth and at a lower speed
   (C) closer to Earth and at a lower speed
   (D) farther from Earth and at a higher speed

101. Assume that a piece of space debris is in a circular orbit at a distance *r* above Earth's surface. If Earth's radius is *R* and the period of the orbit is *T*, what is the speed in orbit of the space debris?

   (A) $\dfrac{2\pi R}{T}$

   (B) $\dfrac{2\pi(R + r)}{T}$

   (C) $\dfrac{2\pi r}{T}$

   (D) $\dfrac{T}{2\pi r}$

102. A curve with a radius of 80 m is banked (angled with the horizontal) at 10°. Suppose that an ice storm hits, and the curve is covered with ice so that it is effectively frictionless. What provides the centripetal force for the car to make the turn?

   (A) the weight of the car
   (B) a component of the friction force perpendicular to the road
   (C) a component of the normal force
   (D) inertia

103. A string that is 1.2 m long will break under a force of 120 N. It is used to spin a 2 kg stone in a vertical circle. Which of the following equations can be used to determine the maximum speed of the stone (without breaking the string)?

(A) $\dfrac{mv^2}{1.2} = mg$

(B) $120 - mg = \dfrac{mv^2}{1.2}$

(C) $mg - mv = 120$

(D) $120 = \dfrac{mv^2}{1.2}$

104. An object with a mass of 2,000 kg moves with a constant speed of 20 m/s on a circular track with a radius of 100 m. What is the magnitude of the acceleration of the object in m/s^2?

(A) 400
(B) 80
(C) 40
(D) 4

105. A car goes around a curve of radius r at a constant speed v. Then it goes around a curve of radius $2r$ at speed $2v$. What is the centripetal acceleration of the car as it goes around the second curve, compared to the first?

(A) the same
(B) twice as great
(C) four times as great
(D) The acceleration cannot be determined without knowing the mass of the car.

106. A stone with a mass of 2 kg is attached to a strong string and whirled in a vertical circle of radius 0.2 m. At the exact bottom of the path, the speed of the stone is 4 m/s. Calculate the tension in the string at this point.

(A) 84 N
(B) 64 N
(C) 32 N
(D) 20 N

107. The radius of the path of an object in uniform circular motion is doubled. For its speed to remain the same, the centripetal force on the object must be

(A) one fourth as much as before
(B) half as much as before
(C) the same as before
(D) twice as great as before

108. An object traveling in a circle at constant speed has

(A) a constant velocity
(B) an inward radial acceleration
(C) an outward radial acceleration
(D) a constant tangential acceleration

109. Consider two satellites in circular orbits around Earth but at different distances from Earth. Which of the following statements is true regarding the centripetal accelerations of the satellites?

(A) Both experience the same centripetal acceleration.
(B) The object nearer to Earth experiences the greater centripetal acceleration.
(C) The object farther from Earth experiences the greater centripetal acceleration.
(D) It depends on the masses of the satellites, which are not known.

CHAPTER 4

Linear Momentum

Conservation Laws

110. An object has a mass of quantity m and a momentum of quantity p. If the momentum of the object doubles, its kinetic energy is

(A) the same
(B) half as much
(C) twice as much
(D) four times as much

111. Which of the following correctly expresses change in velocity?

(A) $\Delta p / \Delta t$
(B) $F \Delta t$
(C) $ma / \Delta t$
(D) $\Delta p / m$

112. On an air track, a 2 kg cart moving at 1 m/s to the right collides with a 1 kg cart moving at 3 m/s to the left. After the collision, the 2 kg cart is moving at 2 m/s to the left. What is the velocity of the 1 kg cart after the collision?

(A) 1 m/s to the right
(B) 1 m/s to the left
(C) 3 m/s to the right
(D) 2 m/s to the left

113. Object A, which is moving to the right at speed $2v$, collides head-on and totally inelastically with an identical object B moving to the left at speed $4v$. What occurs after the collision?

(A) Object A moves to the right at v and Object B moves to the left at $2v$.
(B) Object A moves to the right at $2v$ and Object B moves to the left at v.
(C) The objects move together to the right at speed v.
(D) The objects move together to the left at speed v.

114. Two skaters stand face to face on the ice. Skater 1 has a mass of 40 kg, and skater 2 has a mass of 50 kg. They push off one another and move in opposite directions. What is the ratio of skater 1's speed to skater 2's speed?

(A) 1:1
(B) 1:2
(C) 4:5
(D) 5:4

115. A cart rolls across a level floor and strikes a wall elastically at 10 m/s. In a second trial, the cart strikes the wall at 20 m/s. Assuming that the contact time between the cart and the wall is the same in both cases, compare the force the cart exerts on the wall in the second trial to the force in the first trial.

(A) the same
(B) half as much
(C) twice as much
(D) four times as much

116. A cart on a level air track is moving at $+2$ m/s when it strikes and connects to a stationary cart of the same mass. What is the final velocity of the connected carts?

(A) $+4$ m/s
(B) $+2$ m/s
(C) $+1$ m/s
(D) -1 m/s

117. An experiment is set up with motion sensor A at one end of an air track and motion sensor B at the other end. Chart A shows Velocity as a Function of Time for cart A, which has a mass of 1 kg and moves away from sensor A, and chart B shows Velocity as a Function of Time for cart B, which also has a mass of 1 kg and moves away from sensor B and toward cart A. What is the force exerted by the carts on each other?

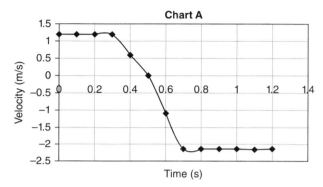

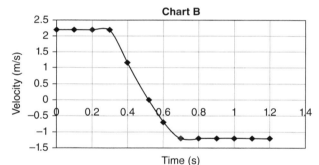

(A) 5.0 N
(B) 8.5 N
(C) 11.0 N
(D) 12.5 N

Impulse and Force

118. The rate at which momentum changes is

   (A) impulse
   (B) kinetic energy
   (C) force
   (D) acceleration

119. The graph shows the force exerted on a tennis ball during a collision with a tennis racket.

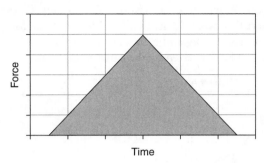

The area between the plot line and the time axis represents

(A) the acceleration of the tennis ball while it is in contact with the racket
(B) the change in momentum of the tennis ball when it hits the racket
(C) the change in velocity of the tennis ball when it hits the racket
(D) the work done by the tennis ball on the racket when it hits the racket

120. A car moving at a speed v is brought to rest in time t by a force F_1. To stop the car in one half the time ($\frac{1}{2}t$), what force F_2 is required?

(A) Force F_2 must be twice as large as F_1.
(B) Force F_2 must be half as large as F_1.
(C) Force F_2 must be one fourth as large as F_1.
(D) The forces required to stop the car are the same in both situations.

121. When automobiles have to stop quickly, injury to occupants can be reduced by using air bags. What is the primary mechanism by which an air bag reduces injury?

(A) An air bag increases the time it takes to stop the person, so the force on the person is less.
(B) An air bag increases the distance over which the person comes to a stop, so the acceleration is larger.
(C) An air bag is soft, so it absorbs the force of the impact.
(D) An air bag applies a force on the person in the opposite direction from the force that the car is exerting on the person, so the net force on the person is less.

122. The graph represents the collision of an object of mass 0.25 kg with a wall. Determine the magnitude of the change in velocity of the object during the impact.

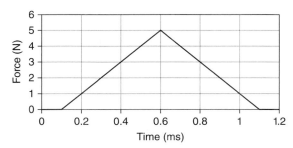

(A) 10 m/s
(B) 1.0 m/s
(C) 0.01 m/s
(D) 0.001 m/s

123. A baseball is thrown toward a target at a speed v and exerts a force F on the target when it collides with it. What is the force exerted on the target if the speed of the baseball is doubled on the second throw (assuming an elastic collision with the target)?

(A) ½F
(B) F
(C) 2F
(D) 4F

Elastic and Inelastic Collisions

124. Which of the following properties are conserved in a totally inelastic collision of two objects, in the absence of external forces on the system of objects?

(A) only momentum
(B) only kinetic energy
(C) both momentum and kinetic energy
(D) neither momentum nor kinetic energy

125. Which of the following statements is NOT always true for change in linear momentum of a system?

(A) There is a change in the velocity of the system.
(B) A net external force must be exerted on the system.
(C) The center of mass of the system changes position.
(D) Either or both the magnitude and direction of momentum change.

126. Which of the following statements is always true for inelastic collisions, assuming there is no external force applied in the direction of motion?

(A) Momentum is conserved, but kinetic energy is not conserved.
(B) Kinetic energy is conserved, but momentum is not conserved.
(C) Both momentum and kinetic energy are conserved.
(D) Energy is not conserved, but the objects exchange velocities during the collision.

127. In the illustration, a particle of mass m_1 moving at speed v along the x axis collides elastically with a stationary particle that has a mass of m_2. After the collision, the mass m_1 is moving at speed v_1 at an angle θ above the x axis and mass m_2 is moving at speed v_2 at angle ϕ below the x axis.

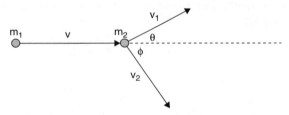

If the two masses are equal and there are no external forces exerted on the system of particles, then

(A) speed v_1 must equal speed v_2
(B) angle θ must equal angle ϕ
(C) $\theta + \phi$ must equal $90°$
(D) speed v must equal $v_1 + v_2$

128. During an inelastic collision, kinetic energy of the system is lost, because kinetic energy

(A) is changed to other forms of energy
(B) must decrease as momentum increases
(C) cannot be conserved during any collision
(D) decreases whenever a force is applied to a system

129. When two moving objects of equal mass collide head-on and elastically, they will

(A) simultaneously come to a stop
(B) exchange velocities during the collision
(C) each have the same velocity after the collision as before the collision
(D) move off at right angles to each other after the collision

130. A photon of light collides with a stationary electron. Using conservation of linear momentum and conservation of mass-energy principles, what is the expected result?

(A) The electron recoils with kinetic energy K and a photon with a longer wavelength is produced.
(B) The electron recoils with kinetic energy K and a photon with a shorter wavelength is produced.
(C) The electron recoils with kinetic energy K and the photon retains its previous speed and wavelength after the collision.
(D) The electron remains stationary and the photon rebounds from it with a shorter wavelength.

131. You are given several small objects, all of the same mass, to throw at an upright block of wood in order to knock it over. To have the best chance of accomplishing this, you will choose

(A) a small dart, thrown at the top of the block so that it sticks in the wood
(B) a small dart, thrown at the bottom of the block so that it does not stick
(C) a small, elastic rubber ball thrown at the base of the block so that it bounces
(D) a small, elastic rubber ball thrown at the top of the block so that it bounces

132. A rubber ball drops from a height of 2 m onto a concrete floor and rebounds to a height of 1 m. What is the coefficient of restitution between the ball and the floor?

(A) 0.25
(B) 0.50
(C) 0.70
(D) 0.90

133. In an experiment, students launch a ball with velocity v_o so that it hits a force sensor horizontally. The sensor registers the force, F, and the time of contact, t. Which of the following expressions could be used to determine the final velocity of the ball of mass m after it collides elastically with the sensor?

(A) $\quad v = \dfrac{Ft}{m} + v_o$

(B) $\quad v = \dfrac{Ftv_o}{m}$

(C) $\quad v = \dfrac{mF}{v_o t}$

(D) $\quad v = \dfrac{Fm}{t} + v_o$

134. A small rocket is fired into the air and lands 30 m forward from the launch site. The rocket is fired a second time at the same velocity and angle. This time, the rocket splits into two pieces at the peak of its motion. The first piece lands on the ground 27 m forward from the launch site. Where would the second piece, which has half the mass of the first piece, land?

(A) 24 m forward from the launch site
(B) 30 m forward from the launch site
(C) 33 m forward from the launch site
(D) 36 m forward from the launch site

135. In the illustration, ball 1, rolling on a level, frictionless table, strikes an identical stationary ball 2, which takes the path shown in the illustration after the collision. What would be the path of ball 1 after the collision?

(A) →
(B) ↙
(C) ↗
(D) Ball 1 is stationary after the collision.

136. A ball is dropped onto the floor from height h and bounces with velocity $-v$ after it hits the floor. The coefficient of restitution between the ball and the floor is 0.5 (the magnitude of the ratio of the ball's velocity after it returns from the floor to its velocity before it hits the floor). If the ball is then dropped from height $4h$, what is its velocity after it hits the floor the second time, assuming the coefficient of restitution is the same?

(A) ½v

(B) v

(C) $2v$

(D) $4v$

137. Two carts have the same mass. Cart A, moving to the right on a track at 6 m/s, collides elastically with cart B, moving to the left on the track at 4 m/s. What are the velocities of cart A and cart B after they collide?

(A) Cart A is moving to the left at 5 m/s, and cart B is moving to the right at 5 m/s.

(B) Cart A is moving to the left at 6 m/s, and cart B is moving to the right at 4 m/s.

(C) Cart A is moving to the left at 4 m/s, and cart B is moving to the right at 6 m/s.

(D) The two carts move together to the right at 5 m/s.

138. A nickel sliding on a smooth surface collides elastically and head-on with a second nickel that is stationary. What is the motion of the nickels after the collision?

(A) The first nickel stops where the second nickel had been sitting, and the second nickel moves off in a straight line with the first nickel's velocity.

(B) The first nickel bounces back and moves backward in a straight line with velocity equal to the negative of its initial velocity.

(C) Both nickels move forward along a line, with the first nickel moving more slowly than the second nickel.

(D) Both nickels move ahead along trajectories that are perpendicular to each other.

139. A nickel sliding on a smooth surface with momentum mv collides elastically and head-on with a second nickel that is stationary. Explain what happens to the nickels in terms of force.

(A) The first nickel stops where the second nickel had been sitting, because the force the second nickel exerts on the first nickel changes the momentum from mv to zero.

(B) The first nickel bounces back and moves backward in a straight line with velocity equal to the negative of its initial velocity, because the force the second nickel exerts is equal to $2mv$.

(C) Both nickels move forward along a line, with the first nickel moving more slowly than the second nickel, because the first nickel exerts more force on the second nickel, causing a large change in momentum.

(D) Both nickels move ahead along trajectories that are perpendicular to each other, because the force is along the line of motion of the first nickel.

140. Two spring-loaded carts are in contact with each other, with springs loaded, on an elevated section of track, as in the illustration.

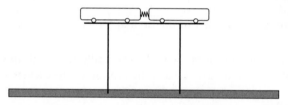

Cart A has twice the mass of cart B. When the spring is released,

(A) cart A moves horizontally with greater velocity and hits the ground first

(B) cart B moves horizontally with greater velocity and hits the ground first

(C) cart B moves horizontally with less velocity and hits the ground first

(D) cart B moves horizontally with greater velocity and the carts hit the ground at the same time

141. An object with a mass of 2 kg moving north at 5 m/s collides totally inelastically with an object having a mass of 4 kg that is moving west at 10 m/s. What is the result of this collision?

(A) The 4 kg object moves south at 5 m/s and the 2 kg object moves east at 10 m/s.

(B) A 6 kg object moves southeast at 50 m/s.

(C) A 6 kg object moves southeast at about 40 m/s.

(D) A 6 kg object moves northwest at about 40 m/s.

142. In the laboratory, a 1 kg cart moving to the right on a track at 2 m/s collides inelastically with a 2 kg cart moving to the left at 2 m/s. After the collision, the 1 kg cart is moving to the left at 2 m/s, and the 2 kg cart stops. Determine the loss to thermal energy during this collision.

(A) 3.0 J
(B) 4.0 J
(C) 12.0 J
(D) 18.0 J

143. In the laboratory, a 1.5 kg cart moving to the right on a track at 2 m/s collides totally inelastically with a 2.0 kg cart moving to the left at 2 m/s. Determine the loss to thermal energy during this collision.

(A) 0.2 J
(B) 4.5 J
(C) 6.4 J
(D) 12 J

144. In an experiment, a small block slides down a track and hits a second, identical block at the edge of a desk 1 m above the floor. The first block is moving horizontally when it hits the stationary block, and the two collide off-center. As a result, the two blocks hit the floor moving in different directions. The first block hits the floor a distance of 0.5 m at an angle of 35° from the center line (a line along the original trajectory of the first block), and the second block hits the floor a distance of 0.25 m at an angle of 55° from the center line. What was the speed of the first block when it hit the second block on the track?

(A) 0.51 m/s
(B) 1.2 m/s
(C) 2.2 m/s
(D) 4.4 m/s

145. In an experiment, a small block slides down a smooth track and hits
a second, identical block at the edge of a desk. The first block is moving
horizontally when it hits the stationary block, and the two collide
off-center. As a result, the two blocks hit the floor moving in different
directions. Which of the following statements can be used to determine
the speed of the moving block before the collision and the speeds of the
two blocks immediately after the collision?

(A) Linear momentum is conserved during the collision, and kinetic
energy is conserved after the collision.
(B) Both linear momentum and kinetic energy are conserved in all three
dimensions.
(C) Linear momentum is conserved during the collision and after the
collision until the blocks hit the floor.
(D) Linear momentum is conserved during the collision but is not
conserved as the blocks fall to the floor.

146. A firecracker with a mass of 6 g is sitting on top of a level table. The firecracker explodes into three pieces, with masses 1 g, 2 g, and 3 g. All the pieces move at the same speed in different directions. (This won't happen often!) Which of the following illustrations shows possible velocity vectors for the three pieces?

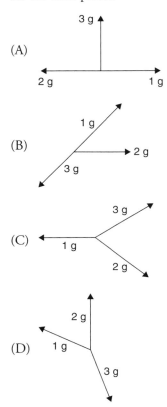

(A)

(B)

(C)

(D)

Torque and Equilibrium

Systems of Forces and Translational Equilibrium

147. In which of the following situations must the net force on the object be zero?

(A) A box is sliding down a frictionless ramp after being released at the top of the ramp.

(B) A satellite is moving at constant speed in a circular orbit.

(C) A box is sliding at constant speed across a level surface.

(D) A hammer is falling to the surface of the moon after being released by an astronaut.

148. Three tension wires are attached to the top of a fence post so that each wire makes a 60° angle when attached to the ground so that the fence post remains stationary. Wire 1 has a tension of 1,000 N and is attached to the east side of the post. Wire 2 has a tension of 2,000 N and is attached to the north side of the post. Which of the following equations could be used to calculate the tension in Wire 3?

(A) $T \cos 60° = \sqrt{(1{,}000 \cos 60°)^2 + (2{,}000 \cos 60°)^2}$

(B) $T = \sqrt{(1{,}000)^2 + (2{,}000)^2}$

(C) $T \cos 45° = \sqrt{(1{,}000 \sin 60°)^2 + (2{,}000 \cos 60°)^2}$

(D) $T \cos 45° = \sqrt{(1{,}000)^2 + (2{,}000)^2}$

149. A box that weighs 10 N is sitting on a ramp that is angled at 30° above horizontal. What is the friction force of the ramp on the box in newtons?

(A) 10
(B) 10 cos 30°
(C) 10 sin 30°
(D) 10 tan 30°

150. A ladder has a mass of 6 kg and is 2 m long. As shown in the illustration, the ladder remains stable against a frictionless wall with its bottom end 1 m from the base of the wall. Rank the following: the weight of the ladder (W), the normal force of the wall on the ladder (N_W), the normal force of the floor on the ladder (N_F), and the friction force of the floor on the ladder (f).

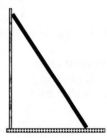

(A) $W > N_F > N_W > f$
(B) $(W = N_F) > (f = N_W)$
(C) $W > (f = N_F) > N_W$
(D) $(W = f) > (N_F = N_W)$

151. An object is attached to a spring and set into oscillation. The system is in equilibrium

(A) at its amplitude, when the instantaneous velocity is zero
(B) when it is moving at its greatest speed
(C) when its displacement is maximum
(D) when its instantaneous acceleration is maximum

152. A Ping-Pong ball is dropped from the top of a building. As it falls, it will reach terminal velocity when

(A) the air drag force becomes greater than the weight of the ball
(B) the vertical forces on the ball reach equilibrium, so that acceleration will be zero
(C) the force accelerating the ball reaches its maximum
(D) the final velocity of the ball is zero

153. An oscillating pendulum is considered to be in translational equilibrium at the lowest point in its motion. Which of the following statements must be true?

(A) The tension in the pendulum string must be equal to the weight of the pendulum bob.

(B) The horizontal force accelerating the pendulum at the bottom of its swing must be equal to the air drag force on the pendulum bob.

(C) The tension in the pendulum string must be equal to *mg* times the sine of the angle from which the pendulum bob was released to start the motion.

(D) The tension in the pendulum string must be equal to the weight of the pendulum bob plus the centripetal force due to the pendulum's motion.

154. In order for a sled to slide at constant speed down an icy hill,

(A) the friction force backward must be equal to the inertial force propelling the sled forward

(B) the friction force must be zero, since there is no force propelling the sled forward

(C) there must be a friction force equal in size to the gravitational force component directed down the hill

(D) there must be no friction force in this situation

Torque, Systems of Torques, and Rotational Equilibrium

155. A force of 100 N is applied to a wheel, as shown in the illustration. The radius of the wheel is 20 cm, and the radius of the axle is 5 cm. For the wheel to rotate at constant speed, determine the magnitude and direction of the friction torque exerted on the axle.

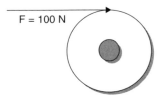

(A) 1.25 N·m clockwise

(B) 1.25 N·m counterclockwise

(C) 20 N·m clockwise

(D) 20 N·m counterclockwise

156. Several meter sticks are stacked on the edge of a table so that the top meter stick is entirely beyond the edge of the table, as shown in the illustration.

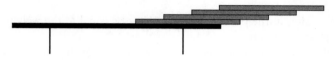

In order for this to occur,

(A) the center of the top stick must be above the stick below it
(B) the center of each stick must be above the table
(C) the center of mass of the entire system of sticks must be at the edge of the table
(D) the left end of the top stick must be directly above the edge of the table

157. When a car is driving across the pavement, which of the following statements best explains what causes the car to move forward?

(A) As the wheels roll, they exert a forward force on the pavement to cause the car to move forward.
(B) The friction force from the pavement on the tires is forward.
(C) The normal force of the pavement on the tires produces a torque that causes the tires to roll.
(D) As the wheels roll forward, they exert a forward force on the car.

158. The diameter of a car's steering wheel is 30 cm, and the diameter of a truck's steering wheel is 40 cm. Assuming that your applied force is the same for both steering wheels, by what percentage does your applied torque increase if you are driving the truck rather than the car?

(A) 10
(B) 15
(C) 25
(D) 33

159. An acrobat performs the "trick" of walking on a loose board laid on top of a flat roof so that one third of the board's length extends beyond the edge of the roof. If the length of the board is 12 ft, the mass of the board is 20 kg, and the mass of the acrobat is 60 kg, how far beyond the edge of the roof can he stand safely on the board?

(A) 3 ft
(B) 2.5 ft
(C) 1 ft
(D) 8 in

160. The distance of a bicycle pedal from its axle is about 18 cm. If a bicycle rider with a mass of 50 kg exerts all of her weight on the pedal, what is the approximate torque applied at the point where the pedal is farthest forward and horizontal?

(A) 50 N·m
(B) 100 N·m
(C) 500 N·m
(D) 1,000 N·m

161. The distance from the elbow to the clenched fist of a person is 30 cm. If the person slowly lifts a 5 kg object from horizontal by bending at the elbow, what is the torque exerted at the elbow?

(A) 10 N·m
(B) 15 N·m
(C) 100 N·m
(D) 150 N·m

162. In the illustration, the rod is 1 m long and has a mass of 200 g. The pivot is 20 cm to the left of the center of the rod. The object on the left end of the rod has a mass of 1 kg, and the object on the right end has a mass of 500 g. What is the net torque on the rod?

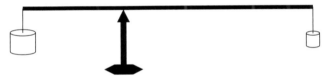

(A) 0.9 N·m clockwise
(B) 3.5 N·m clockwise
(C) 3.5 N·m counterclockwise
(D) 20 N·m counterclockwise

163. For an object or system to be in equilibrium,

(A) the object or system must be stationary
(B) the net force on the object or system must equal zero
(C) the net torque on the object or system must equal zero
(D) both the net force and net torque on the object or system must equal zero

Refer to the illustration for questions 164 and 165.

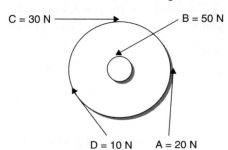

C = 30 N   B = 50 N

D = 10 N   A = 20 N

164. The illustration shows a top view of a wheel and axle system, with forces A, B, C, and D applied at a tangent in each case. The radius of the wheel is 10 cm, and the radius of the axle is 2 cm. What is the net torque on the wheel?

(A) 1 N·m clockwise
(B) 1 N·m counterclockwise
(C) 10 N·m clockwise
(D) 10 N·m counterclockwise

165. The illustration shows a top view of a wheel and axle system, with four forces applied to it so that the forces produce torques. Each force is assumed to be applied on a tangent to either the wheel or the axle. The wheel has a radius of 0.3 m, and the axle has a radius of 0.1 meter. If the wheel and axle system has a rotational inertia of 4 kg·m², what is the angular acceleration of the system?

(A) 0.25 rad/s² clockwise
(B) 0.50 rad/s² counterclockwise
(C) 1.0 rad/s² clockwise
(D) 2.0 rad/s² counterclockwise

166. In the illustration, a fulcrum is placed at a point one third of the length of a thin rod from its left end, a 6 kg mass is attached to the left end of the rod, and a 2 kg mass is attached to the right end.

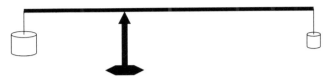

To produce rotational equilibrium, a third mass (1 kg) should be attached

(A) to the left end of the rod
(B) halfway between the fulcrum and the right end of the rod
(C) halfway between the fulcrum and the left end of the rod
(D) to the right end of the rod

167. A bridge, supported by two piers, one at each end, is 20 m long and has a mass of 20,000 kg. A 2,000 kg car is sitting on the bridge 5 m from the center. How much force is each pier exerting upward to support the bridge?

(A) 200,000 N and 20,000 N
(B) 150,000 N and 70,000 N
(C) 110,000 N and 110,000 N
(D) 105,000 N and 115,000 N

168. Two laboratory masses hang from the uniform meter stick in the illustration: a mass of 800 grams at the 15 cm mark and a mass of 350 grams at the 70 cm mark. The meter stick balances horizontally on a pivot placed at the 35 cm mark. What is the mass of the meter stick?

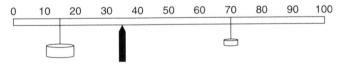

(A) 100 g
(B) 125 g
(C) 200 g
(D) 250 g

169. The meter stick in the illustration has a mass of 0.5 kg. With a 1 kg laboratory mass hanging 0.25 m from the top end, the meter stick remains stable against a frictionless wall with its bottom end 0.50 m from the base of the wall. What is the friction force exerted on the stick by the floor?

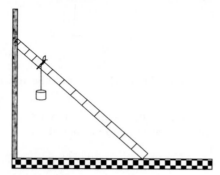

    (A) 3 N
    (B) 6 N
    (C) 8 N
    (D) 9 N

170. A screwdriver that is 12 cm long is used to pry open the lid of a paint can. The person doing this applies a downward force of 100 N at the handle end of the screwdriver and supports the screwdriver on the edge of the can 1 cm from the screwdriver's tip. What is the force required to lift open the paint can without the screwdriver?

    (A) 120 N
    (B) 1,100 N
    (C) 2,000 N
    (D) 11,000 N

171. In the illustration, a wire with tension T helps support a horizontal wooden beam with mass M that has a sign of mass m attached to its end. The beam has a length L and is attached to the wall so that the wire makes a 40° angle. Which of the following expressions could be used to determine the tension in the wire?

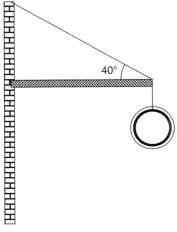

(A) $T \sin 40° = Mg + mg$
(B) $mgL + Mg(\frac{1}{2}L) = T(L \sin 40°)$
(C) $mgL + Mg(\frac{1}{2}L) = T(L \cos 40°)$
(D) $T \cos 40° = Mg + mg$

172. The ladder in the illustration has a mass of 6 kg and is 2 m long. The ladder is stable against a frictionless wall with its bottom positioned 1 m from the base of the wall. Determine the normal force exerted by the wall on the ladder.

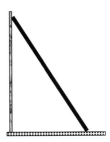

(A) 7 N
(B) 10 N
(C) 13 N
(D) 17 N

173. A meter stick with a mass of 100 g balances horizontally when a pivot is placed at the middle (on the 50 cm mark). When an unknown object is placed at the 80 cm mark, the pivot must be moved to the 60 cm mark for the system to balance. What is the mass of the unknown object?

(A) 10 g
(B) 50 g
(C) 100 g
(D) 200 g

174. A student is attempting to construct a mobile that balances various objects on sticks so that it is in equilibrium. In the illustration, each stick is uniform, is 40 cm long, and has a mass of 10 grams; the distance of an attachment from the center of the stick is noted. Determine the mass of the last object that can be attached to the mobile to make it balance.

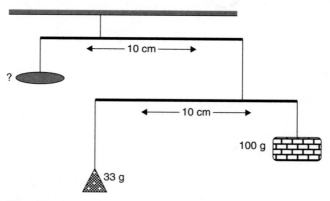

(A) 40 g
(B) 200 g
(C) 2,000 g
(D) 4,000 g

175. In the illustration, three objects are suspended from a thin horizontal rod with a pivot. Object 1 has a mass of 1 kg, object 2 has a mass of 2 kg, and object 3 has a mass of 3 kg. The distances given in the answers are measured from the pivot to the point where each object is attached to the rod. Which of the following arrangements would result in a balanced system?

	Object 1	Object 2	Object 3
(A)	1.0 m	0.5 m	0.5 m
(B)	1.0 m	0.5 m	2.0 m
(C)	2.0 m	1.0 m	0.5 m
(D)	2.0 m	2.0 m	2.0 m

CHAPTER 6

Work, Energy, and Power

Kinetic Energy

176. An object is dropped from a height of 10 m above the ground. What is the ratio of the kinetic energy of the object when it has fallen halfway to its kinetic energy just before it hits the ground?

(A) 2:1
(B) 1:1
(C) 1:2
(D) 1:4

177. A pendulum is pulled back and released from a position 0.2 m higher than its position at the bottom of its swing. What is the speed of the pendulum bob as it moves through the equilibrium position at the bottom of its swing after it is released?

(A) 0.5 m/s
(B) 1 m/s
(C) 1.5 m/s
(D) 2 m/s

178. What happens to the kinetic energy of a space vehicle moving in circular orbit around Earth when the vehicle transfers into an orbit farther from the center of Earth?

(A) Its kinetic energy increases, because the vehicle now has less gravitational potential energy.
(B) Its kinetic energy increases, because more work must be done by gravity to keep it in the higher orbit.
(C) Its kinetic energy decreases, because the vehicle does not move as fast in its orbit when it is farther from Earth.
(D) Its kinetic energy decreases, because the gravitational potential energy is less, and they must remain equal to each other.

179. A 0.5 kg rock is thrown at a speed of 5 m/s horizontally from the top of a building 20 m tall. What is the kinetic energy of the rock when it hits the ground?

(A) 6.3 J
(B) 106 J
(C) 112 J
(D) 160 J

180. An automobile with a mass of 2,000 kg accelerates from a speed of 10 m/s to a speed of 20 m/s in a time period of 6 s. What is the increase in kinetic energy of the vehicle during this time period?

(A) 1,000 J
(B) 6,000 J
(C) 20,000 J
(D) 300,000 J

181. An electron is accelerated from rest to a speed of 6×10^6 m/s by an electric potential difference of 12 volts. Determine the kinetic energy of the electron after the acceleration.

(A) 7.2×10^6 eV
(B) 12 eV
(C) 3.6×10^6 eV
(D) 9.6×10^6 eV

182. Which of the following is NOT a unit that could be used to measure kinetic energy?

(A) joule
(B) erg
(C) electron volt
(D) watt

183. Which of the following illustrations could be the plot of Kinetic Energy as a Function of Time for an object thrown horizontally from the top of a building?

(A)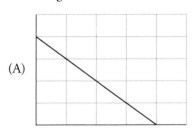

(B)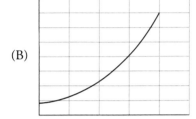

(C)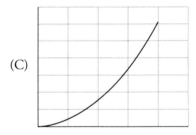

(D)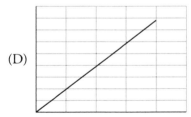

184. A block with a mass of 2 kg is moving at a speed of 3 m/s when it slides horizontally off a roof that is 4 m above the ground. The kinetic energy of the block just before it hits the ground is approximately

(A) 9 J
(B) 20 J
(C) 80 J
(D) 90 J

185. A 2 kg ball that is dropped from a height of 4 m loses 10% of its mechanical energy to thermal energy when it hits the floor. What is the kinetic energy of the ball just after it rebounds from the floor?

(A) 48 J
(B) 64 J
(C) 72 J
(D) 88 J

186. Which of the following could be the plot of Kinetic Energy as a Function of Height above the Ground for an object thrown horizontally from the top of a building?

(A)
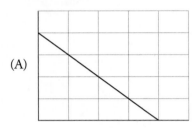

(B)
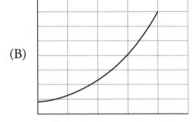

(C)
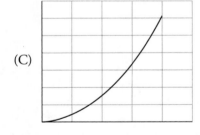

(D)
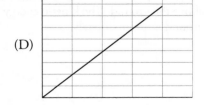

Gravitational Potential Energy

187. A rock with mass m is thrown horizontally at a speed v from the top of a building of height h. What is the kinetic energy of the rock just before it hits the ground?

(A) mgh
(B) $\frac{1}{2}mv^2$
(C) $mgh - \frac{1}{2}mv^2$
(D) $\frac{1}{2}mv^2 + mgh$

188. In the illustration, two objects of unequal mass (20 g and 30 g) are suspended by a string over a pulley. Assuming negligible masses for the pulley and string, determine the change in gravitational potential energy of the smaller object (with respect to Earth) after the system is released and the larger object moves downward a distance of 0.1 meter.

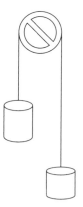

(A) 10 J
(B) 20 J
(C) 0.02 J
(D) 0.01 J

189. What is the ratio of the magnitude of the gravitational potential energy of an Earth-object system when the object is on the surface of Earth to the gravitational potential energy of the same system when the object is two Earth radii above the surface?

(A) 2:1
(B) 3:1
(C) 4:1
(D) 9:1

190. As Earth moves closer to the sun in its orbit (toward perihelion), the gravitational potential energy of the Earth-sun system is

(A) greater, since the two objects are closer together and gravitational forces are greater

(B) greater, since the speed of Earth is greater and both potential energy and kinetic energy increase

(C) less, since kinetic energy is greater and the sum must be constant

(D) less, since the two objects are closer and both potential energy and kinetic energy must decrease

191. The gravitational potential energy of a system of two particles is equal to U. In a second system, the mass of each particle is twice as great and the distance between their centers is half as great. What is the gravitational potential energy of the second system in terms of U?

(A) $\frac{1}{2}U$

(B) $2U$

(C) $4U$

(D) $8U$

Spring Potential Energy

192. A 40 g object is attached to a spring with spring constant $k = 200$ N/m. Compare the potential energy of the spring-object system when the spring is extended 0.01 m beyond the equilibrium position to the system's potential energy when the spring is extended twice as far, to 0.02 m beyond equilibrium.

(A) 1:1

(B) 1:2

(C) 1:4

(D) 1:16

193. A flexible plastic ruler on the top of a table is flexed horizontally a distance of 5 cm, and a 0.1 kg rock is placed against it. When the ruler is released and the rock is propelled off the edge of the table, it is determined that the rock has a speed of 2 m/s. Determine the elastic constant, k, of the ruler.

(A) 8 N/m

(B) 16 N/m

(C) 80 N/m

(D) 160 N/m

194. The graph shows data for amplitude as a function of time for an object with a mass of 0.5 kg oscillating on a spring. At which of the following times is the spring potential energy at a maximum?

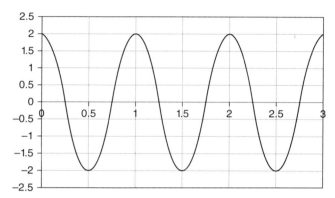

(A) $t = 0.25$ s
(B) $t = 0.50$ s
(C) $t = 1.75$ s
(D) $t = 2.75$ s

195. A spring attached to an object with a mass of 2 kg oscillates according to the equation

$$x(t) = (0.4\ m)\cos 10\ t$$

Determine the elastic constant of the spring.

(A) 10 N/m
(B) 20 N/m
(C) 100 N/m
(D) 200 N/m

196. A spring is placed on a horizontal, frictionless surface and compressed a distance of 0.1 m from its rest position with a ball of mass 0.1 kg placed at its end. When the spring is released, the ball leaves the spring traveling at 10 m/s. What is the spring constant?

(A) 50 N/m
(B) 100 N/m
(C) 500 N/m
(D) 1,000 N/m

Conservative and Nonconservative Forces

197. Which of the following statements is true regarding nonconservative forces?

(A) The gravitational force is nonconservative, because it increases on an object as the object moves closer to Earth's center.

(B) The gravitational force is nonconservative, because the path taken by an object is always in the same direction as the gravitational force exerted on the object.

(C) The friction force is nonconservative, because mechanical energy is converted to thermal energy.

(D) The friction force is nonconservative, because work done by friction is always independent of the path taken.

198. A ball is placed on a ramp and allowed to roll to the bottom onto a table. The velocity of the ball is determined by how far the ball lands from the edge of the table on the floor below. The kinetic energy at the bottom of the ramp is significantly less than the gravitational potential energy change from the top to the bottom of the ramp. What is most likely the reason for this discrepancy?

(A) the work done by the gravitational force on the ball

(B) the work done by the normal force on the ball

(C) the work done by the friction force on the ball

(D) the transfer of thermal energy to the ball from the ramp

199. A 2 kg object slides 30 m down a snow-covered (frictionless) hill to a point that is 10 m lower on the hill. What is the work done by the gravitational force on the object?

(A) 20 J

(B) 60 J

(C) 200 J

(D) 600 J

Conservation of Energy and Work-Energy Theorem

200. The graph displays data for a force applied to a spring. How much work is done on the spring by the applied force in extending the spring a distance of 2 m?

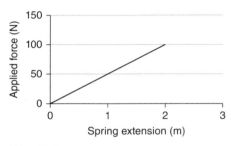

(A) 50 J
(B) 100 J
(C) 200 J
(D) The work cannot be determined without knowing the elastic constant of the spring.

201. A 1,000 kg car is moving at a constant speed of 10 m/s on a level, circular track with a radius of 50 m. How much work is done by the centripetal force on the car (in this case, the friction between the tires and the road) when the car makes one loop on the track?

(A) 50,000 J
(B) 20,000 J
(C) 2,500 J
(D) No work is done by the centripetal force.

202. Which of the following expressions correctly describes the work done *by friction* on a box of mass m sliding across a level floor if the coefficient of friction between the box and floor is μ and the distance the box moves is d?

(A) $\mu m d$
(B) $-\mu m g d$
(C) $\mu m g d$
(D) $-\mu g d$

203. A box of mass m is being pushed a distance d across a level surface at constant speed. In which of the following cases would the most work be done by a force F on the box?

(A) The force F is horizontal and parallel to the floor.
(B) The force F is at a 30° angle to the floor.
(C) The force F is at a 45° angle to the floor.
(D) The force F is at a 60° angle to the floor.

204. On a curved, level roadway with a radius of 100 m, the suggested speed limit is 25 mph (approximately 10 m/s). To safely negotiate the curve at the posted speed, what must the coefficient of friction be between a car's tires and the road?

(A) 0.1
(B) 0.2
(C) 0.3
(D) 0.4

205. An arrow moving at 10 m/s is stopped by a target. If the arrow has a mass of 250 g and penetrates 4 cm into the target, what is the force exerted by the arrow on the target?

(A) 1,250 N
(B) 425 N
(C) 310 N
(D) 25 N

206. A ball with a mass of 250 g is thrown horizontally at a speed of 4 m/s from the top of a platform that is 10 m high. What is the speed of the ball when it hits the ground?

(A) 4 m/s
(B) 8 m/s
(C) 11 m/s
(D) 15 m/s

207. A box with a mass of 6 kg and initially moving at 2 m/s slides a distance of 1 m across a rough floor to a stop. Which of the following values best estimates the coefficient of friction between the box and the floor?

(A) 0.05
(B) 0.1
(C) 0.2
(D) 0.4

208. Students set up a box race, in which two boxes are allowed to slide down a ramp so that they are moving at the same speed when they reach the floor. The boxes are identical, except that box A contains one book and box B is filled with books so that its mass is 10 times the mass of box A. The distance each box travels across the floor after leaving the ramp is compared, so that the box that travels the farthest is declared the winner. Which box will win the competition?

(A) Box A
(B) Box B
(C) It will be a tie; that is, the boxes will travel the same distance across the floor.
(D) The outcome cannot be determined without knowing the mass of the contents of each box.

209. The graph shows data for amplitude as a function of time for an object with a mass of 0.5 kg oscillating on a spring. During which of the following time intervals does the spring do the largest magnitude of net work on the object attached to it?

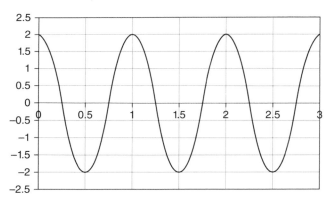

(A) $t = 0$ to $t = 0.5$ s
(B) $t = 0$ to $t = 1.0$ s
(C) $t = 2.5$ to $t = 2.75$ s
(D) $t = 1.0$ to $t = 1.5$ s

210. A horizontal spring with a spring constant of 200 N/m is placed on a horizontal surface and attached at one end to a wall. A block with a mass of 0.5 kg is used to compress the spring a distance of 5 cm. If the mass of the spring is negligible and the coefficient of friction between the block and the surface is 0.02, determine the speed of the block at the moment it loses contact with the spring.

(A) 1 m/s
(B) 0.5 m/s
(C) 0.1 m/s
(D) 0.02 m/s

211. Students want to determine the spring constant of a spring in a small pop-up toy, as shown in the illustration. They assume that the mass of the small plastic top of the toy is negligible. When the students put a 20 g glob of putty on the toy, then push the toy down 1 cm and release it, the spring causes the toy to move an upward distance of 8 cm above its equilibrium position. This is just one trial in a larger set of trials using varying amounts of putty. Using a preliminary calculation from this trial, what would the students predict for the spring constant?

(A) 80 N/m
(B) 160 N/m
(C) 320 N/m
(D) 480 N/m

212. What is the work done in placing a satellite of mass m in orbit at a distance R from Earth's center?

   (A) The work is equal to the weight of the satellite plus the kinetic energy of the satellite.
   (B) The work is equal to the gravitational potential energy of the satellite at that altitude above Earth's surface.
   (C) The work is equal to the gravitational potential energy of the satellite plus the centripetal force necessary to keep the satellite in orbit at that altitude.
   (D) The work is equal to the change in gravitational potential energy of the satellite from the surface to that altitude plus the change in kinetic energy of the satellite.

213. In which of the following cases has a person done the most work on the system described?

   (A) moving a 20 kg box at constant speed across a surface with a coefficient of friction of 0.05, using a force of 10 N for a distance of 10 m
   (B) lifting a 20 kg box onto a shelf that is 2 m high
   (C) holding a 20 kg box 2 m above the floor for 10 minutes
   (D) pushing a 20 kg box across a frictionless surface to accelerate it from rest to 5 m/s

214. An 11 lb bowling ball (with a mass of about 5 kg) is dropped from a height of 1 meter onto a floor. If the dent the ball makes in the floor is about 1 cm deep, estimate the average force the ball exerted on the floor.

   (A) 50 N
   (B) 250 N
   (C) 2500 N
   (D) 5,000 N

Power

215. A 2,000 kg automobile accelerates from rest to a speed of 40 m/s in 20 s. What is the average power, in kilowatts, produced by the automobile during this time interval?

   (A) 10 kW
   (B) 20 kW
   (C) 40 kW
   (D) 80 kW

216. If a lightbulb uses 40 watts of power for an hour, what is the energy used by the bulb?

(A) 40 J
(B) 240 J
(C) 3,600 J
(D) 144,000 J

217. In which of the following cases has a person generated the most power?

(A) moving a 20 kg box at constant speed across a surface with a coefficient of friction of 0.05, using a force of 10 N for a distance of 10 m in a time of 20 s
(B) lifting a 20 kg box onto a shelf that is 2 m high in a time of 2 s
(C) holding a 20 kg box 2 m above the floor for 10 minutes
(D) pushing a 20 kg box across a frictionless surface to accelerate it from rest to 5 m/s in 10 s

218. An average force of 0.2 N is exerted on a 2 kg object to accelerate it from a speed of 2 m/s to 3 m/s in a time interval of 10 s. Determine the average power generated.

(A) 0.5 W
(B) 2.0 W
(C) 5.0 W
(D) 20.0 W

219. A 10 kg object is moving at a constant velocity of 4 m/s on a level surface. If the coefficient of friction between the object and the surface is 0.2, calculate the constant power required to keep the object moving.

(A) 40 W
(B) 80 W
(C) 160 W
(D) 1600 W

220. Experimental data in the chart shows the total energy used by a device as a function of time. What is the average power consumption of this device from $t = 0$ to $t = 10$ s?

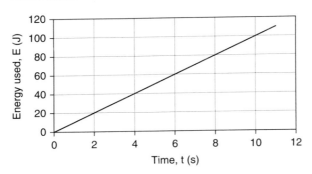

(A) 5 W
(B) 10 W
(C) 500 W
(D) 1,000 W

CHAPTER 7

Thermodynamics

Zeroth Law

221. A small metal cube with a temperature of 308 K is placed in contact with a much larger cube of the same metal with a temperature of 290 K. Assuming no loss of energy to the environment around the cubes, which of the following statements is true regarding the transfer of energy that takes place?

(A) The smaller cube will undergo a greater change in temperature than the larger cube.

(B) After a long time, the final temperature of both cubes will be 299 K.

(C) The smaller cube will contain more internal energy than the larger cube after the two cubes reach an equilibrium temperature.

(D) The smaller cube will actually transfer more energy to the larger cube than the larger cube transfers to the smaller one.

222. A 1 kg block of metal at 200 K is brought into contact with a 3 kg block of the same metal at 300 K. Assuming no loss of energy to the environment around the blocks, which of the following statements is true regarding the temperatures of the blocks after a long time has passed?

(A) The final temperature of each block will be 250 K, because the blocks will reach thermal equilibrium.

(B) The temperatures of the two blocks will be the same, so all molecules will have the same average speed.

(C) The temperatures of the two blocks will be the same, so all molecules will have the same average kinetic energy.

(D) The final temperatures of the blocks can only be the same if the two blocks are made of the same materials.

First Law and Conservation of Energy

223. During an isothermal process involving an ideal gas, the pressure of the gas is doubled. Which of the following statements is true?

   (A) The volume remains constant.
   (B) The temperature also doubles.
   (C) The volume and temperature of the gas also double.
   (D) The temperature remains constant.

224. In a sealed, rigid container of an ideal gas held at constant volume, one would expect

   (A) pressure to increase as temperature increases
   (B) the average kinetic energy of molecules to decrease as pressure increases
   (C) the internal energy of molecules to decrease as temperature increases
   (D) pressure to decrease as temperature increases

225. According to the first law of thermodynamics (the law of conservation of energy for thermodynamic systems), an increase in the temperature of a system during an adiabatic process is due to

   (A) heat added to the system to increase the temperature of molecules
   (B) work done by the molecules of the system in expanding themselves
   (C) work done by an external force on the system, increasing the kinetic energy of molecules
   (D) heat transferred from one part of the system to another

226. An engine receives 475 J from a heat reservoir at 750 K and rejects 315 J to the cold reservoir at 250 K. Determine the actual efficiency and the theoretical maximum Carnot efficiency for this engine.

	Actual	**Carnot**
(A)	33.7%	66.7%
(B)	16.5%	50.0%
(C)	66.7%	66.7%
(D)	50.8%	75.0%

227. How much heat must be added or removed to allow 2 moles of an ideal gas to expand isothermally from 1 m^3 to 3 m^3?

   (A) An amount equal to the work done by the gas must be removed.
   (B) An amount equal to the work done by the gas must be added.
   (C) An amount equal to the product of pressure and volume must be added.
   (D) No heat must be added or removed: $Q = 0$.

228. A rigid container of an ideal gas is heated so that the absolute temperature of the gas doubles while the volume remains constant. The molecules of the gas

(A)   increase in pressure, so they do more work on the walls of the container
(B)   have twice as much internal energy
(C)   must give off energy, since they cannot expand
(D)   have twice the average speed as before

229. An ideal gas at pressure P, volume V, and temperature T undergoes an isothermal process that changes the pressure to $2P$. What is the new volume of the gas?

(A) $\frac{1}{2}V$
(B) V
(C) $2V$
(D) $4V$

230. A system of ideal gas molecules contains 2 moles of gas. Eighty joules of work is done in compressing the gas as the gas gives off 25 J of energy. Then the gas is allowed to expand, doing 40 J of work on its surroundings. What is the net change in internal energy of the gas as a result of these processes?

(A) $+145$ J
(B) -15 J
(C) $+15$ J
(D) $+45$ J

231. Which of the following statements is always true regarding change in internal energy (U) of a system of an ideal gas?

(A)   Internal energy will increase if work is done on the system during an isobaric process.
(B)   Internal energy will decrease if work is done by the system during an isovolumetric process.
(C)   Internal energy will increase if heat is added to the system and work is done on the system.
(D)   Internal energy will increase if heat is added during an isothermal process.

Second Law and Entropy

232. Chamber X, a very large reservoir of gas at a temperature of 400 K, comes into thermal contact with chamber Y, a very large reservoir of gas at 300 K. During a certain time interval, 500 J of heat transfers from chamber X to chamber Y. Which of the following statements is true regarding entropy in this situation?

(A) The entropy change of chamber X is greater than the entropy change of chamber Y.
(B) The entropy change of chamber Y is greater than the entropy change of chamber X.
(C) The entropy changes of chambers X and Y are equal.
(D) Once the chambers come to equilibrium, there has been no net change in entropy.

233. Two isolated chambers of an ideal gas are in thermal contact with each other, Chamber X at a higher temperature T_1 and chamber Y at a lower temperature T_2. If heat is transferred directly from Chamber X to Chamber Y,

(A) the amount of heat transferred out of Chamber X is greater than the heat transferred into Chamber Y
(B) the magnitude of change in entropy of each chamber is the same
(C) the magnitude of change in entropy of Chamber X is greater than the magnitude of change in entropy of Chamber Y
(D) the magnitude of change in entropy of Chamber X is less than the magnitude of change in entropy of Chamber Y

Thermal Energy Transfer (Conduction, Convection, and Radiation)

234. The thermal conductivity of water is 0.609 W/m·C°, of oil 0.145 W/m·C°, and of alcohol 0.202 W/m·C°. Students are designing a container to maintain a constant temperature of a beaker of boiling water inside the container. The students decide to set the beaker into a liquid bath. With which of the following actions would the students be most successful in keeping the water boiling?

(A) Set the beaker into oil at 90°C.
(B) Set the beaker into alcohol at 80°C.
(C) Set the beaker into water at 90°C.
(D) Set the beaker into water at 80°C.

235. Which of the following methods of energy transfer is due to the motion of fluids of varying densities?

(A) conduction
(B) convection
(C) radiation
(D) insulation

236. A hot liquid can be cooled more quickly by stirring it with a silver stick. Which of the following actions would be even more effective in cooling the liquid?

(A) Replace the stick with one twice as long and half the diameter.
(B) Replace the stick with one half as long and twice the diameter.
(C) Replace the stick with one twice as long and twice the diameter.
(D) Replace the stick with one half as long and half the diameter.

237. The rate at which heat flows by conduction from a hot chamber to a cold chamber through a steel rod may be increased by

(A) substituting a rod with the same dimensions but made of a material with higher specific heat
(B) decreasing the temperature of the hot chamber and increasing the temperature of the cold chamber
(C) substituting a shorter steel rod of the same diameter
(D) substituting a thinner steel rod of the same length

238. One method of heat transfer is radiation, which is transfer of energy by electromagnetic waves. This radiation is sometimes called

(A) gamma radiation
(B) infrared radiation
(C) visible light
(D) ultraviolet radiation

239. Which of the following statements describes the mechanism at the molecular level that causes the handle of a metal spoon placed into a kettle of very hot soup to become too hot to touch?

(A) The molecules in the end of the spoon in the soup begin to move faster as they gain energy from the soup, so those molecules move to the handle of the spoon, exciting other molecules in the handle of the spoon—making the handle feel hotter to the touch.

(B) The molecules in the end of the spoon in the soup absorb radiation from the hot soup that is transmitted as thermal energy to the handle of the spoon.

(C) The molecules in the end of the spoon in the soup move farther apart as they gain energy from the soup, making that end of the spoon less dense. As molecules from the handle move to the other end of the spoon to balance out the density, the handle becomes less dense and thus feels hotter.

(D) The molecules in the end of the spoon in the soup have more kinetic energy as they gain energy from the soup. They are moving faster and collide more often with molecules near them, giving them kinetic energy, and so on, until the molecules in the handle have higher kinetic energy too.

240. A solid door is made of a material with a thermal conductivity of 0.1 W/m·C° and has the dimensions 2 m × 1 m × 2 cm thick. The inside temperature is 70°C, and the outside temperature is 20°C. Determine the rate of heat transfer through the door.

(A) 10 J/s
(B) 140 J/s
(C) 200 J/s
(D) 500 J/s

Thermal Expansion

241. Which of the following quantities does NOT normally increase with an increase in temperature?

(A) electrical resistance
(B) the speed of sound in air
(C) the density of a gas
(D) the pressure of a gas at constant volume

242. At room temperature, a brass ball has the same diameter as the inside opening of a brass ring, so the ball just barely fits through the ring. What happens if the ball and ring are heated together to a much higher temperature?

(A) The ball gets larger while the inside diameter of the ring gets smaller.
(B) The ball gets larger while the inside diameter of the ring gets larger.
(C) The ball gets larger while the inside diameter of the ring remains constant.
(D) The ball's diameter remains constant while the inside diameter of the ring increases.

243. A metal ruler is made of a material that has a coefficient of linear expansion of $12 \times 10^{-6}/C°$. If the ruler is heated from $70°C$ to $100°C$, by what percentage does the length of one centimeter on the ruler increase?

(A) about 1%
(B) between 0.5% and 1%
(C) between 0.01% and 0.5%
(D) less than 0.01%

244. A square metal plate 10 cm on a side is made of a material that has a coefficient of linear expansion of $10 \times 10^{-6}/C°$. If the plate's temperature is increased from $70°C$ to $80°C$, what is the new area of the plate?

(A) 100.00 cm²
(B) 100.02 cm²
(C) 100.20 cm²
(D) 101.00 cm²

PV Diagrams

245. During which step of the process shown in the graph is work done on the gas?

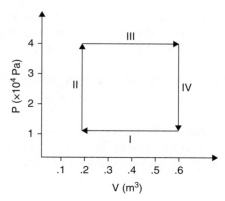

(A) I
(B) II
(C) III
(D) IV

246. A thermodynamic cycle for one mole of an ideal gas is described by the Pressure as a Function of Volume graph. Determine the thermal energy lost or gained by the system during one complete cycle, A-B-C.

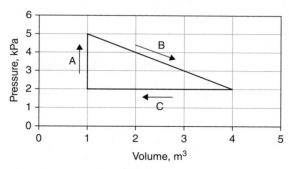

(A) 12,000 J added to the gas
(B) 6,000 J added to the gas
(C) 4,500 J added to the gas
(D) 20,000 J lost by the gas

247. The Pressure as a Function of Volume graph describes a cycle for a thermodynamic process A-B-C for an ideal gas. Pressure is measured in kPa, and volume in cubic meters. In step AB of the process, 78 J of energy are added while volume is held constant. In step BC, the gas remains at constant temperature and 50 J of energy are removed from the system. In step CA, 20 J of energy are removed. How much work is done by the gas in step BC?

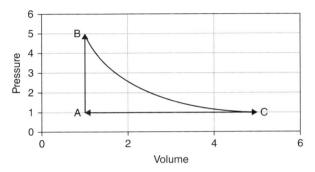

(A) 48 kJ
(B) 24 kJ
(C) 12 kJ
(D) 8 kJ

Refer to the diagram for questions 248 and 249.

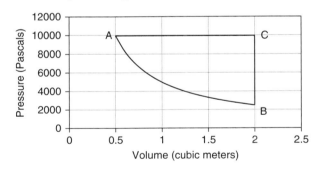

248. The diagram illustrates the pressure and volume changes for two moles of an ideal gas as it is taken through a cycle from state A to B to C and back to A. Which of the following most closely estimates the net work during the cycle?

(A) 10,000 J
(B) 6,000 J
(C) 2,000 J
(D) No net work is done during the cycle shown.

249. Two moles of an ideal gas are taken through a cycle from state A to B to C and back to A, as shown in the diagram. Which of the following statements correctly describes individual steps in the cycle?

(A) AB is isothermal, and BC is isovolumetric.
(B) CA is isothermal, and BC is isobaric.
(C) AB is adiabatic, and CA is isobaric.
(D) AB is isothermal, and BC is isobaric.

250. The pressure/volume graph describes a thermodynamic process A-B-C for an ideal gas in which step BC is isothermal. The term *adiabatic* describes a process in which no heat is transferred into or out of a system. Which of the steps in the process could be adiabatic?

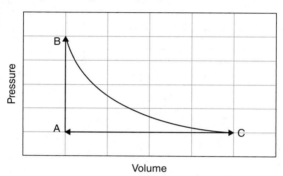

(A) AB, because no work is done on or by the gas
(B) BC, because temperature remains constant
(C) CA, because there is no pressure change and thus no work is done on or by the gas
(D) None of these steps could be adiabatic.

CHAPTER 8

Periodic Motion, Mechanical Waves, and Sound

Harmonic Motion and Wave Functions

251. At what point during the oscillation of a pendulum is the acceleration of the pendulum bob equal to zero?

(A) at the amplitude of the swing
(B) at the bottom of the swing
(C) halfway between the amplitude and bottom of the swing on the way down
(D) halfway between the amplitude and bottom of the swing on the way up

252. An object attached to a spring is displaced by 4 cm and released to set it into oscillation with a period of time T. Then the same object on the same spring is displaced by 8 cm and set into oscillation again. What is the period of the second oscillation?

(A) T
(B) $T/2$
(C) $2T$
(D) $4T$

253. A simple pendulum oscillates with a period of T seconds. The length of the pendulum is doubled, and the mass attached to the pendulum is doubled. What will be the new period of the pendulum's oscillation?

(A) $\frac{1}{4}T$
(B) $\frac{1}{2}T$
(C) $\sqrt{2}\,T$
(D) $2T$

254. An object is attached to a spring and set into motion, oscillating vertically. Which of the following statements is true regarding the motion of the object at the lowest point of its oscillation?

(A) The object's velocity and acceleration are equal to zero.
(B) The object's velocity and displacement from equilibrium are both maximum.
(C) The object's acceleration is equal to zero and displacement is a maximum.
(D) The object's velocity is equal to zero and displacement is a maximum.

255. As a simple harmonic oscillator decreases in amplitude under the influence of friction,

(A) period and frequency both decrease
(B) total mechanical energy and frequency both decrease
(C) total mechanical energy decreases and period increases
(D) total mechanical energy decreases and frequency remains constant

256. A 1 kg mass oscillates on a spring with a period of 0.5 s and an amplitude of 4 m. Which of the following equations describes the position of the oscillating mass as a function of time?

(A) $x(t) = 2 \cos 2\pi t$
(B) $x(t) = 4 \cos 4\pi t$
(C) $x(t) = 2 \cos \pi t$
(D) $x(t) = 4 \cos 0.5\pi t$

257. The equation for a certain harmonic oscillator is $x(t) = (2.5 \text{ m}) \sin 4t$. The amplitude and period of the oscillations are, respectively,

(A) 2.5 m and 0.5π s
(B) 2.5 m and 2π s
(C) 0.3 m and 2π s
(D) 0.3 m and 4 s

Refer to the graph for questions 258 and 259.

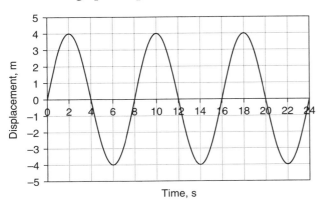

258. The graph plots displacement as a function of time for a mass oscillating on a spring. At what time(s) is the velocity of the oscillating mass equal to zero?

    (A) 6 s and 10 s
    (B) 4 s and 12 s
    (C) $t = 0$ only
    (D) 8 s and 14 s

259. The graph plots displacement as a function of time for a mass oscillating on a spring. At what time are the displacement and acceleration in opposite directions?

    (A) $t = 0$
    (B) $t = 4$ s
    (C) $t = 6$ s
    (D) all of the above

260. A certain wave is produced by the oscillations of particles of a medium in the $+y$ and $-y$ direction, as the wave pulses travel in the $+x$ direction. What type of wave is this?

    (A) transverse
    (B) longitudinal
    (C) compressional
    (D) spherical

261. Sound waves produced in one end of a cardboard tube (point A) move to the ear of a listener at the other end of the tube (point B). As the waves move from A to B inside the tube, which of the following occurs?

(A) Energy is transferred from A to B.
(B) Air molecules are transferred from A to B.
(C) Oscillations of molecules occur perpendicular to a line from A to B.
(D) The frequency of oscillations decreases as the waves move farther in the tube from A to B.

262. As a musician "warms up" a wind instrument to play, the temperature of the air in the instrument increases. What is the result of this change in the fundamental for the instrument?

(A) an increase in frequency and wavelength
(B) an increase in frequency and decrease in wavelength
(C) an increase in wave speed and frequency
(D) an increase in wave speed and decrease in frequency

263. The graph records Position as a Function of Time for two different sound sources; the solid line is source A and the dashed line is source B. Which of the following statements correctly compares the two waves?

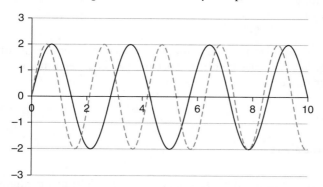

(A) Sound wave A has a higher frequency than sound wave B.
(B) Sound wave A has a higher amplitude than sound wave B.
(C) The two waves undergo constructive interference at about 8.0 s.
(D) The two waves undergo destructive interference at about 4.2 s.

264. In the illustration, there are two small openings on the left spaced 1 mm apart. Waves coming from the left go through the openings in the same phase and produce an interference pattern with a central maximum at point B and a first order maximum at point A. Assuming that point P is the midpoint between the openings, line PB is 10 cm from the opening, and point A is 2 mm from point B, what is a possible wavelength of the waves?

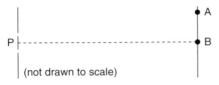

(not drawn to scale)

(A) 0.02 mm
(B) 1 mm
(C) 200 mm
(D) 10 cm

265. The wave diagram of Amplitude (m) as a Function of Time (s) represents two oscillators of the same amplitude but different frequency. The wave for oscillation A is indicated with a solid line, and the wave for oscillation B is indicated with a dashed line. The period of wave A is 2.9 s, and the period of wave B is 2.1 s. At what times would the waves come closest to being in the same phase?

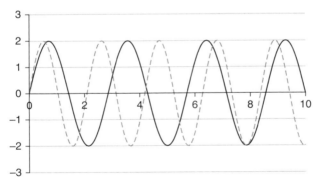

(A) wave A at $t = 0$ and wave B at $t = 1$
(B) wave A at $t = 0.7$ and wave B at $t = 3.7$
(C) wave A at $t = 2.2$ and wave B at $t = 3.7$
(D) wave A at $t = 6.5$ and wave B at $t = 8.3$

Amplitude, Intensity, and Intensity Level

266. A speaker is moved twice as far away from you, but the volume is turned up so that the intensity at the source doubles. What is the resultant intensity of the sound where you sit, compared to what it was before the speaker was moved and the volume adjusted?

(A) half the intensity
(B) one fourth the intensity
(C) twice the intensity
(D) four times the intensity

267. The equation to calculate decibel level for sound is $\beta = 10 \log(I/I_o)$, where I_o is the intensity of the lowest limit of human hearing, 1×10^{-12} W/m². What is the corresponding decibel level of a sound that has an intensity of 1×10^{-10} W/m²?

(A) 2 dB
(B) 10 dB
(C) 20 dB
(D) 40 dB

268. If the sound level in a room increases from 50 decibels to 60 decibels, by what factor has the actual intensity increased?

(A) 2 times
(B) 6 times
(C) 10 times
(D) 100 times

Wave Interference and Harmonics

269. The following graph of Wave Amplitude as a Function of Time shows two waves: a sine function with a dashed line and a cosine function with a solid line. At what time would the superposition of the two waves have a maximum positive value?

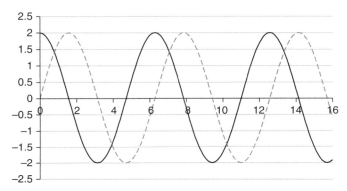

(A) $t = 0$
(B) $t = 7$
(C) $t = 9$
(D) $t = 12$

270. The graph shows two wave pulses, each traveling at a speed of 5 m/s in the direction shown along the x axis. The y axis is amplitude in meters, and the x axis is position in meters. After what time would the superposition of the two waves equal zero?

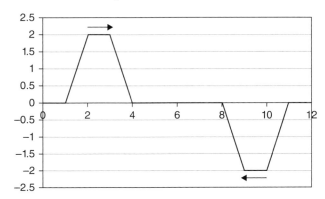

(A) $t = 0.1$ s
(B) $t = 0.2$ s
(C) $t = 0.5$ s
(D) $t = 0.7$ s

271. Two mechanical wave pulses are moving along the x axis toward each other at the same speed. If the pulses are traveling at 2 m/s, at what time after the "snapshot" shown here will the waves superimpose to produce a wave of the greatest amplitude?

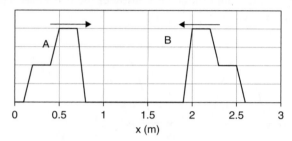

(A) 0.25 s
(B) 0.38 s
(C) 0.75 s
(D) 1.0 s

272. Two speakers output the same tone in the same phase. A person sitting in a chair across the room at the same distance from both speakers hears the tone very well. However, when the person moves the chair to the right so that he is one half meter closer to one speaker than to the other, he is not able to hear the tone well. What is the wavelength of the tone produced by the speakers?

(A) 0.25 m
(B) 0.5 m
(C) 1 m
(D) 1.5 m

273. Blowing across a tube open at both ends produces a musical note. Assuming that the length of the tube is L and the speed of sound in the air inside the tube is v, what is the fundamental frequency of the musical note?

(A) $2L/v$
(B) $4L/v$
(C) $v/4L$
(D) $v/2L$

274. Blowing across a tube open at both ends produces a musical note. If you place your finger over the open end of the tube at the bottom and blow across the top of the tube, a second note is produced. Compare the pitch and frequency of the second note to that of the note produced with the pitch and frequency of the original note.

(A) The second note has a higher pitch and twice the frequency.
(B) The second note has a higher pitch and one half the frequency.
(C) The second note has a lower pitch and twice the frequency.
(D) The second note has a lower pitch and one half the frequency.

275. A tube that is 20 cm long and closed at one end should produce the same fundamental note as

(A) a 10 cm tube open at both ends
(B) a 20 cm tube open at both ends
(C) a 30 cm tube open at both ends
(D) a 40 cm tube open at both ends

276. A guitar string attached at both ends is 40 cm long and produces a fundamental note of frequency 200 Hz when it is plucked. What are the frequencies of the first and second overtones of this string?

(A) 200 and 300 Hz
(B) 100 and 200 Hz
(C) 200 and 400 Hz
(D) 400 and 600 Hz

277. The air column in a tube open at one end and closed at the other end is 0.8 m long and produces a fundamental note of frequency 100 Hz when the tube is struck to set up a standing wave. What are the frequencies of the first two overtones of this tube?

(A) 200 and 300 Hz
(B) 100 and 300 Hz
(C) 200 and 400 Hz
(D) 300 and 500 Hz

278. A tube open at both ends and a tube open at one end and closed at the other end both resonate at a fundamental frequency f. What is the next higher frequency at which each tube will resonate?

	Open Tube	Closed Tube
(A)	f	$2f$
(B)	$2f$	$2f$
(C)	$2f$	$3f$
(D)	$2f$	$4f$

279. A tube that is open at one end and closed at the other end, with a length L, produces a standing wave with a fundamental frequency f. If the tube is cut in half, what is the fundamental frequency of the shorter tube?

(A) $f/4$
(B) $f/2$
(C) $2f$
(D) $4f$

280. A string is stretched between two fixed points, and a standing wave of two complete loops is produced on the string using a frequency generator. Which of the following actions will produce a standing wave of three complete loops on the string?

(A) Decrease the frequency setting on the generator, keeping all other conditions the same.
(B) Replace the string with a thinner string of the same length and tension.
(C) Loosen the string to decrease the tension.
(D) Move the supports apart to increase the distance between the fixed points.

281. Two tuning forks, with frequencies of 256 and 260 Hz, respectively, are struck at the same time. An observer hears six beats per second. What causes this?

(A) constructive and destructive interference of superimposed waves
(B) refraction of the overlapping waves
(C) diffraction of waves through the tuning forks
(D) attenuation and damping of the superimposed waves

282. Three tuning forks have the same frequency. A piece of clay is attached to the top of one tuning fork, which is labeled Y. A second tuning fork is left unchanged and is labeled X. A third tuning fork has a different piece of clay attached to the top and is labeled Z. When X and Y are struck simultaneously, 5 beats per second are produced. When Y and Z are struck simultaneously, 3 beats per second are produced. How does the frequency of tuning fork Z compare to the frequency of tuning fork X?

(A) Tuning fork Z is 3 Hz less than tuning fork X.
(B) Tuning fork Z is 8 Hz less than tuning fork X.
(C) Tuning fork Z is either 8 Hz or 2 Hz less than tuning fork X.
(D) Tuning fork Z is 5 Hz greater than tuning fork X.

283. On a street corner, you are playing middle A (440 Hz) on a saxophone. In the open bed of an approaching pickup truck, a trombone is also playing middle A. You hear a beat frequency of 4 Hz. What frequency do you hear from the trombone and what property of sound waves is being demonstrated in this problem?

Frequency	**Property**
(A) 444 Hz	Doppler effect
(B) 444 Hz	Fundamental frequency
(C) 436 Hz	Doppler effect
(D) 436 Hz	Harmonics

284. Two open plastic pipes produce the same 260 Hz frequency when they are struck. One pipe is sanded so that it is slightly shorter, and the pipes produce 4 beats per second when they are struck at the same time. What is the frequency of the shorter pipe?

(A) 65 Hz
(B) 256 Hz
(C) 264 Hz
(D) 1,040 Hz

285. A clarinet is tuned to play middle C. Which property of the note does NOT change as the clarinet is played and the air becomes warmer inside the instrument?

(A) wavelength
(B) speed
(C) frequency
(D) pitch

Sound Transmission, Doppler Effect, and Ultrasound

286. As sound waves travel in a fluid from a region of higher density to a region of lower density, the waves may change direction. What is the best explanation for this?

(A) diffraction
(B) attenuation
(C) reflection
(D) refraction

287. As sound travels through a medium, its amplitude decreases or is attenuated by scattering and absorption. Attenuation of sound in fluids directly increases with

(A) the density of the medium and the frequency of the sound
(B) the frequency of the sound and the viscosity of the medium
(C) the density of the medium and the speed of sound in the medium
(D) the speed and frequency of the sound

288. Generally speaking, the speed of sound will be highest in air that is

(A) more dense and less elastic
(B) less dense and less elastic
(C) more dense and more elastic
(D) less dense and more elastic

289. Which of the following is an example of sound diffraction?

(A) A car horn sounds less loud as it moves away from you.
(B) You are able to hear a sound from an invisible car horn around the corner of a building.
(C) A fire truck siren sounds higher in pitch when it is moving toward you than when the truck stops.
(D) On a cold night at the ballpark, you see the batter hit a ball and then hear the sound.

290. Ultrasonic sound waves can be transmitted into and reflected from different media, such as human tissue, to identify the structure, based on how strongly the transmitted sound amplitude decreases as a function of distance and frequency. Which of the following is the constant that quantifies this decrease in amplitude in a given material?

(A) the elastic constant
(B) the attenuation coefficient
(C) the coefficient of restitution
(D) the coefficient of linear expansion

291. Which of the following situations will produce the greatest Doppler shift of frequency for the frequency of a siren heard by an observer?

(A) The observer is sitting at an intersection as the siren approaches the intersection from the east at a speed of 30 m/s.

(B) The siren is located at an intersection as the observer is moving away from the intersection toward the west at 30 m/s.

(C) The observer is in a car moving north at 30 m/s toward an intersection as the siren is moving toward the same intersection from the east at a speed of 30 m/s.

(D) The observer is in a car moving north at 30 m/s away from an intersection as the siren is moving toward the same intersection from the south at a speed of 30 m/s.

292. You are driving on a divided highway at 30 m/s and encounter an emergency vehicle with a siren that is emitting a constant frequency. In which of the following situations will you hear the highest frequency from the siren?

(A) The emergency vehicle is behind you, moving in your direction at 40 m/s.

(B) The emergency vehicle is ahead of you, moving away from you at 40 m/s.

(C) The emergency vehicle is ahead of you, moving toward you from the other direction at 40 m/s.

(D) The emergency vehicle is in the lane next to you, moving in the same direction at 30 m/s.

293. Ultrasound can be used to speed up chemical reactions, because the ultrasonic signal

(A) can interact directly with molecules to give them the energy to react

(B) produces local extremes in temperature and pressure, thereby increasing reaction rate

(C) breaks up solids in solutions, thereby increasing reaction rate

(D) Both B and C are possibilities.

294. Which of the following best describes ultrasonic?

(A) sound with a frequency higher than 20,000 Hz

(B) cyclic pressure in a medium with a frequency lower than 20 Hz

(C) supersonic pressure oscillations in a medium

(D) sound that cannot be perceived by humans, due to differences in physical properties

CHAPTER 9

Fluids and Solids

Density and Specific Gravity

295. An irregularly shaped piece of halite (salt) has a mass of 220 g. In order to find its volume without dissolving it, it is submerged in oil, which has a density of 0.80 g/cm³. The sample displaces 100 ml of oil. What is the density of the sample?

(A) 2.8 g/cm³
(B) 2.2 g/cm³
(C) 1.8 g/cm³
(D) 0.45 g/cm³

296. A block of wood is placed in water and floats 60% submerged (and thus 40% above water). When the block is placed in an alcohol that is 90% as dense as water, the block

(A) floats 90% under the surface of the alcohol
(B) floats 67% under the surface of the alcohol
(C) floats 54% under the surface of the alcohol
(D) sinks in the alcohol

297. An object with volume V floats in a fluid with density ρ so that the object is 75% submerged in the fluid. Which of the following correctly expresses the density of the object?

(A) $\dfrac{4\rho}{3}$

(B) $\dfrac{3\rho}{4}$

(C) $\dfrac{\rho}{3}$

(D) $\dfrac{\rho}{4}$

298. A solution is comprised of two liquids that are nonmiscible, that is, they do not dissolve in each other to produce a reduction in total volume. The solution is made of 60 ml of liquid A, which has a specific gravity of 0.5, and 40 ml of liquid B, which has a specific gravity of 0.7. What is the specific gravity of the solution?

(A) 0.58
(B) 0.67
(C) 0.75
(D) 1.2

299. A ball floats half submerged in a liquid. Which of the following statements is true?

(A) The ball's density is the same as the liquid's density.
(B) The buoyant force on the ball is greater than the weight of the ball.
(C) The buoyant force on the ball is less than the weight of the ball.
(D) The ball's weight is equal to the weight of the fluid displaced.

300. A block of a certain material that is insoluble in water sinks when placed in a container of distilled water, then eventually rises to the surface. The block is removed and placed in a second container of distilled water, where the block floats and then eventually sinks. Which of the following is the best explanation for this?

(A) The block has a greater density than distilled water at room temperature.
(B) The first container was filled with hot water.
(C) The first container was filled with cold water.
(D) Both containers initially contain water at room temperature.

301. A rock is tied to a spring scale and lowered into water in a graduated cylinder so that the rock is submerged and the spring scale reads 0.80 N. When the rock goes under water, the water level in the cylinder rises from the 35 ml mark to the 45 ml mark. What is the mass of the rock?

(A) 40 g
(B) 50 g
(C) 80 g
(D) 90 g

302. A ball floats 60% below the surface when placed in water and 70% below the surface when placed in a second liquid. The density of water is 1,000 kg/m³. Which of the following most closely approximates the density of the second liquid?

(A) 550 kg/m³
(B) 600 kg/m³
(C) 850 kg/m³
(D) 1,100 kg/m³

Archimedes' Principle and Buoyancy

303. In the illustration, a bar of metal is suspended under water by two cords. If T is the tension in each cord, W is the weight of the bar in air, and F is the buoyant force of the water on the bar, which of the following equations correctly expresses the forces on the bar of metal?

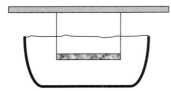

(A) $F = 2T - W$
(B) $2T + F = W$
(C) $W > 2T - F$
(D) $2T = W$

304. A ball with a radius of 2 cm and a mass of 20 g floats in water. What is the buoyant force on the ball?

(A) 0.1 N
(B) 0.2 N
(C) 0.3 N
(D) 0.4 N

305. Water is poured into a U-shaped tube. Oil is poured into one side, and the liquid levels are allowed to come to equilibrium. Using the information given in the illustration, determine the density of the oil.

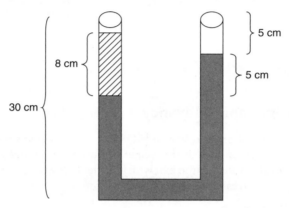

(A) 600 kg/m³
(B) 700 kg/m³
(C) 800 kg/m³
(D) 900 kg/m³

Hydrostatic Pressure and Pascal's Law

306. The density of fresh water is 1,000 kg/m³, and atmospheric pressure is 101 kPa. Determine the absolute pressure at the bottom of a freshwater lake that has a depth of 20 m and a surface area of 21,000 m².

(A) 100 kPa
(B) 200 kPa
(C) 300 kPa
(D) 400 kPa

307. Freshwater lake A has a surface area of 800 m² and a depth of 40 m, and freshwater lake B has a surface area of 1,000 m² and a depth of 20 m. Compare the total pressure at the bottom of lake A with that of lake B.

(A) Lake A has greater pressure at the bottom, because it has a greater depth.
(B) Lake A has greater pressure at the bottom, because it has a greater volume of water.
(C) Lake B has greater pressure at the bottom, because it has a greater surface area.
(D) The two lakes have equal pressure at the bottom.

308. A tank is 8 m tall and has a bottom area of 50 m². It is filled to a depth of 6 m with fresh water. Calculate the absolute pressure at the bottom of the tank.

(A) 81,000 Pa
(B) 101,000 Pa
(C) 161,000 Pa
(D) 181,000 Pa

309. A tank is 8 m tall and has a bottom area of 50 m². It is filled to a depth of 6 m with fresh water. Calculate the fluid force on the bottom of the tank.

(A) 1×10^5 N
(B) 8×10^5 N
(C) 4×10^6 N
(D) 8×10^6 N

310. The average density of sea water is 1,025 kg/m³. Calculate the force, in newtons, on the top of a one-square-meter section of a sunken ship at a depth of 4,000 m.

(A) 1×10^5 N
(B) 4×10^6 N
(C) 4×10^7 N
(D) 1×10^8 N

311. The total fluid pressure on a scuba diver at the bottom of a lake does NOT depend on

(A) atmospheric pressure
(B) the density of the water
(C) water depth
(D) the surface area of the lake

312. An air bubble with a volume of 0.001 m³ is released at a depth of 21 m in a freshwater lake. The volume of the bubble when it reaches the surface is nearest to

(A) 0.001 m³
(B) 0.002 m³
(C) 0.003 m³
(D) 0.004 m³

313. A balloon filled with helium gas will float to the ceiling of a room on Earth. What will happen to the same balloon when released on the surface of the moon?

(A) The gravitational force on the moon is less, so the balloon has less weight and will rise even faster.

(B) Since there is no atmosphere on the moon, the balloon will expand to a larger volume and float more easily than on Earth.

(C) Since there is no air on the moon to provide a buoyant force on the balloon, it will sink to the surface.

(D) Since the surface of the moon is so cold, the balloon will shrink and thus have a lower density.

Fluid Flow and Viscosity

314. A certain pipe carries water at 20°C, delivering 10 m³ per minute. The water is then cooled to 15°C. How does the volume rate of flow compare, and what is the best explanation?

(A) The flow rate will stay the same, because rate of flow does not depend on temperature.

(B) The flow rate will increase, because viscosity increases when temperature is lower.

(C) The flow rate will decrease, because the decrease in viscosity will decrease speed.

(D) The flow rate will decrease, because viscosity increases.

315. Students are performing an experiment to determine the viscosities of various liquids by dropping a small metal sphere into graduated cylinders filled with the liquids, taking measurements, and then using the following equation to determine the viscosity of each liquid.

$$\eta = \frac{2(\Delta\rho)^2 gr^2}{9v}$$

where η is viscosity, $\Delta\rho$ is the difference in densities between the sphere and the liquid, g is 9.8 m/s², r is the radius of the sphere, and v is the speed of the sphere as it falls through the liquid. Water has a viscosity of 0.001 Pa·s and a density of 1,000 kg/m³, and olive oil has a viscosity of 0.1 Pa·s and a density of 900 kg/m³. The metal sphere has a radius of 1 cm and a density of 7,500 kg/m³. How would the ball's speed falling through water approximately compare to its speed falling through olive oil?

(A) The speed is about the same for each liquid.
(B) The ball will fall about 10 times faster through water than through olive oil.
(C) The ball will fall about 100 times faster through water than through olive oil.
(D) The ball will fall about 500 times faster through water than through olive oil.

Continuity Equation

316. Water flows horizontally from a larger pipe with a diameter of 20 cm to a smaller pipe with a diameter of 10 cm. The smaller pipe then curves upward, and the water flows at a level 2 m higher, as in the illustration. If the speed of the water is 4 m/s in the larger pipe, what is the speed of the water in the smaller pipe as it flows at the higher level?

v = 4 m/s   2 m

(A) 8 m/s
(B) 10 m/s
(C) 12 m/s
(D) 15 m/s

317. If you place your thumb over the end of a garden hose of running water, what is the effect on the speed of water flow and the amount of water leaving the hose each second?

(A) The speed of flow and the amount of water flow both increase.

(B) The speed of flow increases and the amount of water flow decreases.

(C) The speed of flow increases and the amount of water flow stays the same.

(D) The speed of flow decreases and the amount of water flow increases.

318. A trough with a semicircular cross section is level-full, with water flowing at a speed of 3 m/s. If the depth of the water at the center of the trough is 0.20 m, what is the approximate volume of water flowing past a given point per hour?

(A) 120 m^3

(B) 680 m^3

(C) 1,400 m^3

(D) 2,200 m^3

Turbulence at High Velocities

319. An increase in which of the following properties of a moving fluid will NOT produce an increase in turbulence of the fluid flow?

(A) the density of the fluid

(B) the diameter of the obstacle encountered in the fluid flow path

(C) the velocity of the fluid flow

(D) the viscosity of the fluid

320. In which of the following situations is blood flow in a vessel most likely to become turbulent?

(A) The blood flows from a vessel of small diameter to a vessel of larger diameter.

(B) The blood flows from a vessel of large diameter to a vessel of smaller diameter.

(C) The blood becomes less dense due to hydration.

(D) The blood becomes more viscous.

Surface Tension

321. Which of the following properties of real fluids are not found in "ideal fluids"?

(A) density and viscosity
(B) viscosity and surface tension
(C) surface tension and density
(D) none of the above

322. Which of the following actions would NOT be effective in reducing surface tension in water?

(A) heating
(B) adding an inorganic salt
(C) adding sugar
(D) adding a surfactant

Bernoulli's Equation

323. The illustration shows an open container of water with a spout 60 cm from the bottom that allows a stream of water to flow out of the container. When the height of water above the spout is 45 cm, what is the speed of the water flowing out of the spout?

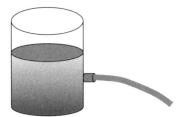

(A) 3.0 m/s
(B) 5.0 m/s
(C) 6.0 m/s
(D) 7.5 m/s

324. The speed of air moving over the top of a thin airfoil, such as an airplane wing, is 50 m/s, and the speed of air moving under the airfoil is 40 m/s. If the area of surface is approximately 30 m², what is the lift force on the airfoil due to the moving air? (Assume the density of air is 1.29 kg/m³.)

(A) 580 N
(B) 1,000 N
(C) 10,200 N
(D) 17,400 N

325. A student wants to determine the speed of water flowing from a garden hose. The student turns the water flow on to maximum and directs the hose straight upward. The water stream travels to a maximum height of 2 m above the spout of the hose. What is the approximate speed of the water?

(A) 2 m/s
(B) 4 m/s
(C) 6 m/s
(D) 8 m/s

326. Bernoulli's equation is a statement of

(A) conservation of mass in fluid flow
(B) conservation of linear momentum in fluid flow
(C) conservation of energy in fluid flow
(D) the property of laminar flow of fluids

327. Air is moving horizontally from a wide pipe of diameter 1 cm at a speed of 2 m/s to a narrow pipe of diameter 0.5 cm. Assuming that the density of air is 1.29 kg/m³ and neglecting change in density due to compression, what is the change in internal pressure of the air?

(A) 10 Pa
(B) 20 Pa
(C) 30 Pa
(D) 40 Pa

Elasticity and Elastic Limit

328. For permanent deformation of an object to occur,

(A) the stress on the object must be proportional to the strain
(B) the stress on the object must be greater than the elastic limit
(C) the strain on the object must be greater than the stress
(D) the stress on the object must produce fracture

329. The graph shows data for Stress as a Function of Strain for a brass rod. What is the closest approximation for elastic limit for this rod?

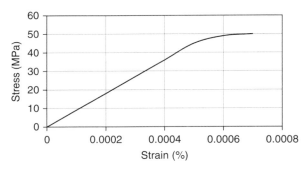

(A) 0.0005%
(B) 0.0007%
(C) 35 MPa
(D) 45 MPa

Shear and Compression of Solids

330. The tension Young's modulus for human bone is 1.6×10^{10} N/m², the compression Young's modulus is 0.94×10^{10} N/m², and the shear modulus is 8.0×10^{10} N/m². What can be concluded from this data?

(A) It takes more force to twist a bone than to stretch the bone the same amount.
(B) It takes more force to stretch a bone than to twist the bone the same amount.
(C) It takes more force to compress a bone than to stretch the bone the same amount.
(D) It takes more force to compress a bone than to twist it the same amount.

331. It is determined that a vertical cylindrical steel rod must support 4 times more weight than previously calculated. Which of the following actions will meet this requirement without causing deformation of the rod?

(A) Replace the rod with a rod that has twice the diameter.
(B) Replace the rod with a rod of the same diameter but four times longer.
(C) Replace the rod with a rod of the same size but with a lower Young's modulus.
(D) Replace the rod with a rod of the same diameter but half as long.

CHAPTER 10

Electrostatics

Charge and Charge Conservation

332. How many electrons are transferred in the process of charging a latex balloon to 1.6×10^{-8} C?

(A) 1×10^{11}
(B) 2.56×10^{-27}
(C) 1×10^{27}
(D) 1×10^{-25}

333. A metal sphere with a charge of $+2Q$ comes into contact with a metal sphere of identical size that has a charge of $-4Q$. The spheres are then separated. What are the charges on the spheres after they are separated?

(A) Both spheres have zero net charge.
(B) Each sphere has a charge of $-2Q$.
(C) Each sphere has a charge of $-Q$.
(D) Each sphere retains its original charge.

334. A negatively charged rod is brought near a second rod that is neutral and suspended by a nonconducting string. The second rod begins to move toward the negative rod, showing attraction of the two rods. After the first rod is removed, the second rod

(A) has no net charge
(B) has a positive net charge
(C) has a negative net charge
(D) is polarized, with one end negative and one end positive

335. A negatively charged rod is brought near a second rod that is neutral and suspended by a nonconducting string. A wire is connected from the second rod to the ground. With the first rod held in place, the ground wire is cut and the first rod is removed. After the first rod is removed, the second rod

(A) has no net charge
(B) has a positive net charge
(C) has a negative net charge
(D) is polarized, with one end negative and one end positive

336. An isolated solid metal sphere that sits on an insulating stand is given a net charge of -10 μC. Which of the following statements best describes the charged sphere?

(A) The net charge will be distributed evenly throughout the volume of the sphere.
(B) The net charge will be distributed evenly over the surface of the sphere.
(C) The net charge will concentrate on the side of the sphere near the insulating stand.
(D) The net charge will be distributed evenly, with half the charge on the outside of the sphere and half the charge on the inside of the sphere.

337. An isolated nonconducting sphere is given a net charge of -10 μC by touching it with a negatively charged rod. Which of the following statements best describes the charged sphere?

(A) The net charge will be distributed evenly throughout the volume of the sphere.
(B) The net charge will be distributed evenly over the surface of the sphere.
(C) The net charge will concentrate on the side of the sphere where the rod touched it.
(D) The net charge will be distributed evenly, with half the charge on the outside of the sphere and half the charge on the inside of the sphere.

Coulomb's Law

338. The electric force between two charged objects is 0.02 N. If each object is given twice its original charge and the objects are located at their original distance from each other, what is the new force?

(A) 0.01 N
(B) 0.02 N
(C) 0.04 N
(D) 0.08 N

339. The electric force between two charged objects is 0.02 N. If the objects are moved four times as far apart, what is the new force?

(A) 0.0012 N
(B) 0.0025 N
(C) 0.0050 N
(D) 0.01 N

340. Four equally charged positive particles are held in position in a square arrangement, so that each side of the square has a length R. What is the net force on an electron placed in the center of the square?

(A) $F = \dfrac{3kq^2}{R^2}$

(B) $F = \dfrac{4kq^2}{R^2}$

(C) $F = \dfrac{\sqrt{2}\,kq^2}{R^2}$

(D) 0

341. The illustration shows three charged particles held in position along a line. What is the net electric force on the particle with charge q_2 due to the other two charges? Let $k = 1/(4\pi\varepsilon_o)$.

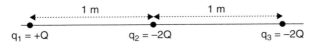

$q_1 = +Q$ 1 m $q_2 = -2Q$ 1 m $q_3 = -2Q$

(A) $6kQ^2$ to the left
(B) $6kQ^2$ to the right
(C) $3kQ^2$ to the left
(D) $3kQ^2$ to the right

342. In a laboratory, an oil droplet carrying a two-electron charge is observed to hover between electrically charged plates so that the electric force upward is equal to the gravitational force downward. Which of the following expressions can be used to determine the mass of the oil droplet?

(A) $m = \dfrac{gE}{2e}$

(B) $m = \dfrac{2eE}{g}$

(C) $m = \dfrac{eE}{g}$

(D) $m = \dfrac{gE}{e}$

343. Two particles, each carrying a net charge of $+6$ μC, are placed on the x axis at $x = -3$ m and $x = +3$ m, as in the illustration. What is the electric force due to the two charges on a particle with a charge of $+6$ μC placed at point P, which is located at position $(0, +3$ m$)$?

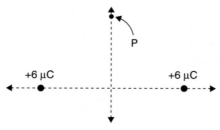

(A) 0.002 N
(B) 0.025 N
(C) 4,200 N
(D) 8,400 N

344. The theoretical distance of an electron (in its ground state) from the proton nucleus of a hydrogen atom is called the Bohr radius, which is approximately 5.29×10^{-11} m. What is the electric force of the proton on the electron at this distance?

(A) 1.5×10^{-17} N
(B) 1.5×10^{-10} N
(C) 9.1×10^{-9} N
(D) 9.1×10^{-7} N

345. The atomic radius of a carbon atom is about 70 pm, or about 70×10^{-12} m. What is the force of the nucleus of a carbon atom (atomic number = 12) on an outer-shell electron at that radial distance?

(A) 1.5×10^{-17} N
(B) 1.5×10^{-10} N
(C) 4.7×10^{-8} N
(D) 5.6×10^{-7} N

Electric Field

346. Two particles, each carrying a net charge of $+6$ μC, are placed on the x axis at $x = -3$ m and $x = +3$ m, as in the illustration. What is the electric field due to the two charges at point P, which is located at position $(0, +3$ m$)$?

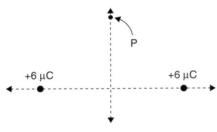

(A) 12 N/C
(B) $6\sqrt{2}$ N/C
(C) 4,200 N/C
(D) 8,400 N/C

347. Determine the electric field at a distance of 2 cm from the center of an object that has a net charge of 2 nC.

(A) 4,500 N/C
(B) 9,000 N/C
(C) 45,000 N/C
(D) 90,000 N/C

348. Four equally charged positive particles are held in position in a square arrangement, so that each side of the square has a length R. What is the net electric field at the center of the square due to the four charges?

(A) $E = \dfrac{4kq}{(\sqrt{2}R/2)^2}$

(B) $E = \dfrac{4kq}{R^2}$

(C) $E = \dfrac{\sqrt{2}kq}{R^2}$

(D) 0

349. Four charged particles—two of charge $+q$ and two of charge $-q$—are held in position in a square arrangement, so that each side of the square has a length R. The two positive charges are held at opposite corners, and the two negative charges are held at opposite corners. What is the net electric field at the center of the square due to the four charges?

(A) $E = \dfrac{4kq}{(\sqrt{2}R/2)^2}$

(B) $E = \dfrac{4kq}{R^2}$

(C) $E = \dfrac{\sqrt{2}kq}{R^2}$

(D) 0

350. An isolated hollow metal sphere has a net positive charge transferred to it. Where is the electric field strongest?

(A) At the exact center of the sphere
(B) Just inside the outer surface of the sphere
(C) Just outside the outer surface of the sphere
(D) At all points halfway from the outer surface to the center of the sphere

Refer to the illustration for questions 351 and 352.

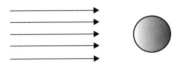

351. An uncharged solid metal sphere is placed into a uniform electric field directed to the right, as shown in the illustration. Which of the following statements best describes what will happen to the sphere?

(A) Since the sphere is uncharged, nothing will happen to it in the field.
(B) Charges in the sphere will separate, with the right side of the sphere more positive.
(C) Charges in the sphere will separate, with the right side of the sphere more negative.
(D) The field will exert a force on electrons, causing them to move away to the right, leaving the sphere with a net positive charge.

352. An uncharged metal sphere is placed into a uniform electric field, as shown in the illustration. Which of the following illustrations best represents the electric field in the region of the sphere after the sphere is placed into the field?

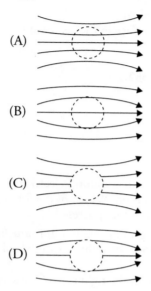

353. The illustration shows two parallel charged metal plates. Which of the following statements is NOT true regarding the situation shown?

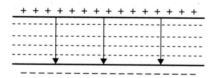

(A) The arrows represent the direction of the electric field between the plates.

(B) The horizontal dashed lines represent equipotential surfaces.

(C) The top plate is at higher electric potential than the bottom plate.

(D) The electric field increases in magnitude moving upward in the diagram.

354. The illustration shows three charged particles held in position along a line. What is the net electric field at point P due to the two charges? Let $k = 1/(4\pi\varepsilon_o)$.

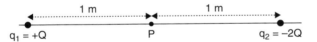

(A) kQ to the left
(B) kQ to the right
(C) $3kQ$ to the left
(D) $3kQ$ to the right

Absolute Potential, Potential Energy, and Potential Difference

355. Assuming that all charges in the illustration have the same magnitude, which of the following combinations of charges would require the greatest amount of work to assemble in the triangular arrangement shown?

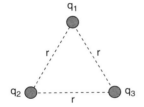

(A) three positive charges
(B) three negative charges
(C) two positive charges and one negative charge
(D) either case in which all three charges have the same sign

356. As the distance from a charge doubles,

(A) the electric field reduces to one half and the electric potential reduces to one half
(B) the electric field remains constant and the electric potential reduces to one half
(C) the electric field reduces to one quarter and the electric potential reduces to one half
(D) the electric field reduces to one quarter and the electric potential reduces to one quarter

357. Which of the following does NOT obey an inverse square law, that is, strength or intensity decreases with the inverse square of distance?

(A) gravitational field
(B) light intensity
(C) electric field
(D) electric potential

358. The two charges in the illustration are held in position on the x axis, with the $+2q$ charge at $x = 3$ and the $-4q$ charge at $x = 6$. At what point on the line is the absolute electric potential equal to zero?

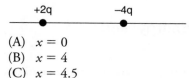

(A) $x = 0$
(B) $x = 4$
(C) $x = 4.5$
(D) $x = 5$

359. Assuming negligible internal resistance in a AA (1.5 V) battery, what is the change in electric potential energy when 0.5 C of charge is transferred between the terminals of the battery?

(A) 0.5 J
(B) 0.75 J
(C) 3.0 J
(D) 4.5 J

360. In the illustration, the arrows represent a uniform electric field of magnitude 100 N/C. A charged particle is moved a distance of 0.02 m from point X to point Y along a path. What is the magnitude of the change in electric potential of the particle, in volts, when it moves from point X to point Y?

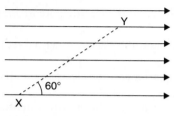

(A) $(100)(0.02)$
(B) $(100)(0.02) \sin 60°$
(C) $(100)(0.02) \cos 60°$
(D) $100/0.02$

Equipotential Lines

361. In the illustration, three positive charges of equal magnitude are held in position in a triangular arrangement. Where could a line be drawn so that every point on the line has the same electric potential due to the three charges?

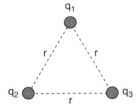

(A) along a line from charge q_1 to charge q_2
(B) along a line from charge q_1 straight down, perpendicular to the line between q_2 and q_3
(C) along a line from the center of the triangle, straight outward, perpendicular to the page
(D) along a closed curve surrounding the three charges

362. In the illustration, two particles carry the same amount of positive charge. Which of the dashed lines could be an electric equipotential line for the two charged particles?

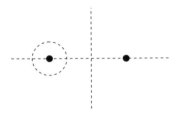

(A) the vertical line that is located halfway between the two charged particles, with every point on the line equidistant from the two particles
(B) the circle around one charged particle, with every point on the circle equidistant from the center of the charged particle
(C) the horizontal line that runs directly through the center of each charge
(D) None of the three lines could be an equipotential line for both charges.

363. Estimate the potential energy of a 3×10^{-6} C charge when it is placed at a distance of 0.01 m from another 3×10^{-6} C charge. (Use 9×10^{9} N·m²/C² for $1/(4\pi\varepsilon_o)$, or Coulomb's constant.)

(A) 8.1 J
(B) 81 J
(C) 810 J
(D) 2.7 MJ

Electric Dipoles

364. In the illustration, an electric dipole is placed in a uniform electric field so that it is free to rotate. In which orientation will the dipole become aligned in the field?

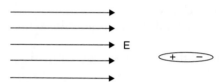

(A) The dipole will align with the positively charged end to the right.
(B) The dipole will align with the positively charged end to the left (as shown).
(C) The dipole will align with the positively charged end toward the top.
(D) The dipole will align with the positively charged end toward the bottom.

365. Which of the following is an example of an electric dipole?

(A) a magnet
(B) Earth
(C) a water molecule
(D) a proton

Gauss's Law

366. A hollow conductive sphere has a net positive charge Q. Two Gaussian surfaces are defined as follows: (A) a spherical Gaussian surface enclosing the sphere, outside the sphere, and (B) a spherical Gaussian surface just inside the surface of the sphere. What is the enclosed charge calculated for each defined Gaussian surface?

(A) Q for surface A and Q for surface B
(B) zero for surface A and zero for surface B
(C) Q for surface A and zero for surface B
(D) zero for surface A and Q for surface B

Refer to the illustration for questions 367 and 368.

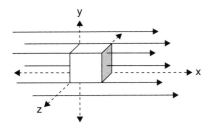

367. A nonconductive, uncharged hollow cube is 2 m on each side. The cube is placed with one corner at the origin into a uniform electric field of strength 100 N/C that extends throughout the region and in the positive x direction, as shown. The sides of the cube extend from $x = 0$ to $x = 2$, from $y = 0$ to $y = 2$, and from $z = 0$ to $z = 2$. What is the net electric flux through the cube?

(A) 0 N·m
(B) 100 N·m in the positive x direction
(C) 100 N·m in the negative x direction
(D) 50 N·m in the positive x direction

368. A nonconductive, uncharged hollow cube is 2 m on each side. The cube is placed with one corner at the origin into a uniform electric field of strength 100 N/C that extends throughout the region and in the positive x direction, as shown. The sides of the cube extend from $x = 0$ to $x = 2$, from $y = 0$ to $y = 2$, and from $z = 0$ to $z = 2$. After the cube is placed into the field, the electric flux at the point (2,1,1) is ϕ to the right out of the cube. The electric flux at the point (0,1,1) is 2ϕ to the right into the cube. What conclusion can be drawn about the contents of the cube?

(A) The cube must be empty, since the flux is to the right.
(B) The cube must contain some sort of negative charge, since the flux to the right is reduced.
(C) The cube must contain some sort of positive charge, since the flux to the right is reduced.
(D) The surface of the cube must be negatively charged.

CHAPTER 11

Electric Circuits

Current, Resistance, and Potential Difference

369. When a net charge of 3.6 μC moves past a given point in 10 ms, what is the electric current?

    (A) 0.36 mA

    (B) 0.36 A

    (C) 3.6 A

    (D) 36 A

370. Which of the following quantities is equivalent to one ampere (A)?

    (A) 1 C/s

    (B) 1 J·s/C

    (C) 1 V·J

    (D) 1 V/s

371. In the circuit diagram, the resistors are connected to an emf of 20 V. Assuming negligible resistance in the wires and in the battery, determine the current in the 3 Ω resistor when the switch is closed.

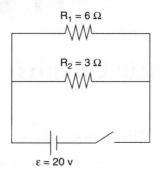

(A) 10 A
(B) 6.7 A
(C) 3.3 A
(D) 2.0 A

372. In the circuit diagram, three identical resistors, each with resistance R, are connected to a battery with potential difference V. When the switch is closed, the current in the resistor on the far right in the diagram could be determined by using which of the following formulas?

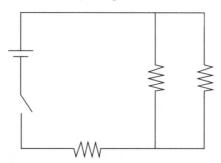

(A) $\dfrac{2V}{3R}$

(B) $\dfrac{V}{3R}$

(C) $\dfrac{4V}{3R}$

(D) $\dfrac{V}{4R}$

373. In a circuit, a 20 Ω resistor and a 30 Ω resistor are connected in series to a 10 V battery. After the switch is closed, what is the electric potential difference in the 20 Ω resistor?

(A) 10 V
(B) 6 V
(C) 5 V
(D) 4 V

Batteries, emf, and Internal Resistance

374. A battery with an emf of 12 V has an internal resistance of 2 Ω. What is the current through the battery when it is connected to an external resistance of 16 Ω?

(A) 0.50 A
(B) 0.67 A
(C) 1.5 A
(D) 2.0 A

375. A battery with an emf of 12 V delivers 10 V to an external circuit when the current in the circuit is 1 A. What is the internal resistance of the battery?

(A) negligible
(B) 0.5 Ω
(C) 1 Ω
(D) 2 Ω

Resistors in Series and in Parallel and Resistivity

376. The circuit in the diagram shows five identical lightbulbs connected to a battery. If each bulb has a resistance of 100 Ω, find the equivalent (total) resistance of the five bulbs.

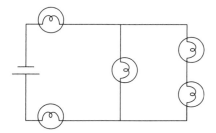

(A) 500 Ω
(B) 270 Ω
(C) 80 Ω
(D) 50 Ω

377. In the diagram, three 100 Ω resistors are connected in a circuit. What is the equivalent resistance of the three resistors?

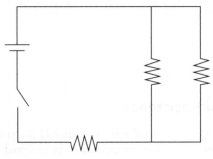

(A) 300 Ω
(B) 200 Ω
(C) 150 Ω
(D) 100 Ω

378. In the diagram, four resistors are connected in a circuit. What is the equivalent resistance of the four resistors?

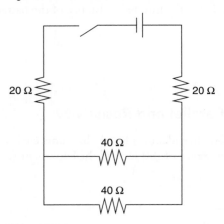

(A) 120 Ω
(B) 100 Ω
(C) 80 Ω
(D) 60 Ω

379. Which of the following statements is true of all combinations of resistors arranged in parallel?

(A) The current splits so that each resistor has the same current.
(B) The potential difference across each branch of the combination is the same.
(C) Both the current and the potential difference are the same in each branch.
(D) The total resistance increases as more resistors are added in parallel.

380. Which of the following formulas correctly expresses the resistivity of a resistor that has resistance R, length L, and cross-sectional area A?

(A) $\rho = \dfrac{RL}{A}$

(B) $\rho = \dfrac{RA}{L}$

(C) $\rho = \dfrac{AL}{R}$

(D) $\rho = \dfrac{R^2L}{A}$

381. Which of the following statements is true regarding the electrical conductivity of a wire?

(A) When an electric potential difference is applied across the metal, the resulting electric field causes electrons to move from one end of the wire to the other.
(B) The electrical conductivity of a wire is proportional to the length of the wire.
(C) Increasing the cross-sectional area of a wire increases the resistance to movement of electrons in the wire, so the conductivity decreases.
(D) All of the above

Capacitors and RC Circuits

382. A parallel plate capacitor stores 100 µJ of energy when charged to an electric potential difference of 20 V. If the capacitor is charged again to a potential difference of only 10 V, what will be the energy stored in the same capacitor?

(A) 200 µJ
(B) 100 µJ
(C) 50 µJ
(D) 25 µJ

383. A 2,000 µF capacitor is charged to 10 V. What is the energy stored in the capacitor?

(A) 0.2 J
(B) 0.1 J
(C) 200,000 J
(D) 100,000 J

384. A 2,000 µF capacitor is charged to 10 V. Without removing any of the charges or changing the plate area or dielectric, the plates are moved apart so that there is twice the distance between them as before. What happens to the energy stored in the capacitor?

(A) Positive work is done in moving the plates apart, so the energy stored in the capacitor increases.
(B) The capacitance increases when the distance between plates increases, so the potential difference between the plates also increases and the energy in the capacitor increases.
(C) Negative work is done in moving the plates apart, so the energy stored in the capacitor decreases.
(D) The capacitance decreases when the distance between the plates increases, so the energy stored in the capacitor decreases.

385. A capacitor is charged to a potential difference of 10 V. Compare the energy stored in the same capacitor if it is charged to 20 V.

(A) The energy is the same in both cases.
(B) There is one half as much energy at 20 V.
(C) There is twice as much energy at 20 V.
(D) There is four times as much energy at 20 V.

386. In the circuit diagram, two capacitors are connected to a 10 V battery. After the capacitors are charged, what are the properties of charge and potential difference for each capacitor?

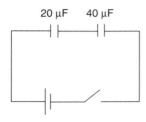

20 µF   40 µF

(A) Both capacitors have the same charge, but the smaller capacitor has twice the potential difference.

(B) Both capacitors have the same potential difference, but the smaller capacitor has half as much charge.

(C) The smaller capacitor has half as much charge and twice the potential difference.

(D) Both capacitors have the same charge, but the smaller capacitor has half the potential difference.

387. A 2,000 µF capacitor and a 4,000 µF capacitor are connected in series in a circuit with a 100 V battery. What is the equivalent capacitance of the two capacitors?

(A) 1,300 µF

(B) 2,000 µF

(C) 3,000 µF

(D) 6,000 µF

388. A 2,000 µF capacitor and a 4,000 µF capacitor are connected in parallel in a circuit with a 100 V battery. What is the equivalent capacitance of the two capacitors?

(A) 6,000 µF

(B) 3,000 µF

(C) 2,000 µF

(D) 1,300 µF

389. A parallel plate capacitor with plate area A and plate separation d and containing a dielectric with dielectric constant κ is charged to a potential difference of 20 V. The capacitor is discharged and the dielectric is replaced with a material that has a dielectric constant of ½κ, without changing A or d. The modified capacitor is then charged again to 20 V. Compare the charge Q_2 stored on the modified capacitor to the charge Q_1 stored on the original capacitor.

(A) $Q_2 = Q_1$
(B) $Q_2 = 2Q_1$
(C) $Q_2 = 4Q_1$
(D) $Q_2 = ½Q_1$

390. The circuit in the diagram consists of a 1 MΩ resistor, a battery with an emf of 20 V, and a 1,000 µF capacitor. The switch is closed, and the capacitor is charged for a very long time. What is the charge on the capacitor?

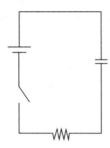

(A) 100 µC
(B) 10,000 µC
(C) 2,000 µC
(D) 20,000 µC

391. The circuit in the diagram consists of two identical 50 Ω resistors, a 100 μF capacitor, and a battery with a potential difference of 10 V. The switch is closed, and the capacitor is charged for a very long time. What is the potential difference across the plates of the capacitor?

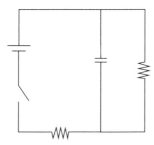

(A) 10 V
(B) 9 V
(C) 5 V
(D) 1 V

Power in Circuits

392. In which of the following actions is the most average power required?
(A) lifting a 5 kg block to a height of 2 m in 2 s
(B) pushing a block across a level surface with a net force of 10 N at a velocity of 3 m/s
(C) changing the kinetic energy of a rolling wheel from 15 J to 55 J in 20 s
(D) burning a lightbulb that has a resistance of 10 Ω using 2 A

393. A 12 V battery is connected to a 4 Ω resistor in a simple series circuit. What is the power dissipated as heat by the resistor?
(A) 48 W
(B) 36 W
(C) 24 W
(D) 12 W

394. In the circuit diagram, what is the total power output of the battery in the circuit?

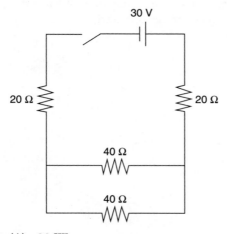

(A) 90 W
(B) 60 W
(C) 45 W
(D) 15 W

Alternating Current and RMS Current and Voltage

395. In the graph, the plots of Current as a Function of Time and Voltage as a Function of Time are superimposed for an alternating current circuit. Which of the following statements is true regarding the circuit?

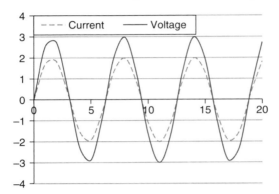

(A) The rms voltage times the rms current is equal to the power output.
(B) The rms voltage and rms current are maxima at the same point in time.
(C) The rms voltage is equal to the maximum voltage divided by $\sqrt{2}$.
(D) All of the above

396. In a small transformer, the input is marked 120 V AC and the output is marked 9 V AC, 350 mA. What is the input current, disregarding power loss to heating?

(A) 14 A
(B) 470 mA
(C) 26 mA
(D) 4.7 A

CHAPTER 12

Magnetic Fields and Electromagnetism

Magnetic Fields

397. The coil in the illustration is made up of wraps of coated wire and is connected to a battery so that it carries an electric current. What is the direction of the magnetic field inside the coil?

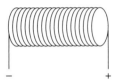

- (A) to the right
- (B) to the left
- (C) in a spiral pattern that follows the coil of wire
- (D) There is no field inside the coil; the field is outside the coil only.

398. A coil of wire with N turns has a radius of R and a current of I. Which of the following actions will increase the strength of the magnetic field inside the coil?

- (A) Reduce the number of turns of wire in the coil.
- (B) Insert an iron rod into the middle of the coil.
- (C) Reduce the current in the coil.
- (D) None of these actions will increase the magnetic field.

399. In the illustration, two parallel wires carry currents I_1 and I_2. In which of the three regions could the net magnetic field due to the wires be equal to zero?

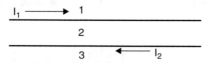

(A) region 1
(B) region 2
(C) region 3
(D) both Region 1 and Region 3

Refer to the illustration for questions 400 and 401.

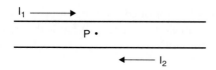

400. In the illustration, two parallel wires have currents of equal magnitude moving in opposite directions. What is the direction of the net magnetic field at point P, which is located equidistant from the wires, due to the currents in the wires?

(A) to the right
(B) into the page
(C) out of the page
(D) There is no net magnetic field at point P.

401. In the illustration, the current in the bottom wire is switched so that the two parallel wires have currents of equal magnitude moving in the same direction. What is the direction of the net magnetic field at point P, which is located equidistant from the wires, due to the currents in the wires?

(A) to the right
(B) into the page
(C) out of the page
(D) There is no net magnetic field at point P.

402. In which of the following cases would a uniform magnetic field B exert the largest magnitude of force on a charged particle?

(A) The charge is $3q$ and is placed stationary in the magnetic field.
(B) The charge is $2q$ and is moving at velocity v directly along the magnetic field lines.
(C) The charge is q and is moving at velocity v perpendicular to the magnetic field line.
(D) The charge is q and is moving at an angle of $60°$ to the direction of the magnetic field.

403. The coil in the illustration has an electric current moving in the direction shown. At which point is the magnetic field strongest?

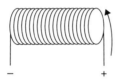

−   +

(A) in the exact center of the coil, midway from each end
(B) midway from each end of the coil, closer to one edge of the coil
(C) at the center of one end
(D) The magnetic field has the same strength at every point inside the coil.

404. In the illustration, a positive charge is placed at rest in the middle of a uniform magnetic field that is directed into the page, in the $-z$ direction. What will be the direction of the subsequent motion of the charge?

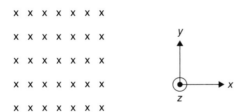

(A) The charge will move upward on the page, in the $+y$ direction.
(B) The charge will move to the right, in the $+x$ direction.
(C) The charge will move into the page, in the $-z$ direction.
(D) The charge will not move.

405. Which of the following statements describes the magnetic field around a long, straight, current-carrying wire?

(A) The magnetic field is along the wire in the same direction as the current and is stronger nearest the wire.

(B) The magnetic field is along the wire in the opposite direction as the current and is stronger nearest the wire.

(C) The magnetic field is in a circular pattern around the wire and is stronger nearest the wire.

(D) The magnetic field is in a helical pattern around the wire and is of uniform strength along the direction that the helix spirals around the wire.

406. Which of the following statements best describes Earth's magnetic field?

(A) Earth's magnetic field may be related to an iron-nickel core and the spin of the planet.

(B) Earth's magnetic field lies along the direction that the north magnetic pole of a compass points.

(C) Earth's magnetic field has its current south magnetic pole in northern Canada.

(D) All of the above

407. In the illustration, two current-carrying wire coils are placed end to end and moved very close to each other. How will the coils affect each other?

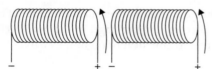

(A) The two coils will attract each other.

(B) The two coils will repel each other.

(C) The two coils will have no effect on each other.

(D) The effect cannot be determined without knowing the size of the current in each coil.

408. The strong magnetic field of a material such as neodymium is due primarily to

(A) how electrons are paired in atoms of the material

(B) the spin nature of electrons in the atom

(C) the alignments of atoms within the material

(D) all of the above

Moving Charges in Magnetic Fields

409. The illustration shows a beam of protons entering a magnetic field at angle *x*. What will be the initial change in direction of the motion of the protons as they enter the field?

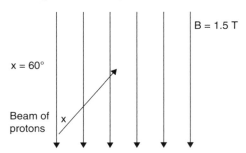

B = 1.5 T

x = 60°

Beam of protons   x

(A) upward on the page
(B) downward on the page
(C) into the page
(D) out of the page

410. The mass of a charged particle can be determined by analyzing its motion as it moves into a magnetic field in a synchrotron. Assume a particle with a charge $+2e$ moving at velocity v into a magnetic field of strength B, perpendicular to the direction of the field. The particle moves in a circular path with a radius R. Which of the following equations can be used to calculate the mass of the particle?

(A) $m = \dfrac{eB}{vR}$

(B) $m = \dfrac{2eB}{vR}$

(C) $m = \dfrac{2eBR}{v}$

(D) $m = \dfrac{eB}{2vR}$

411. In the illustration, a charged particle is propelled from the left, in the $+x$ direction, into a magnetic field. As the particle enters the field, it curves downward on the page, in the $-y$ direction. In what direction would an electric field be added to the magnetic region so that the same charged particle continues straight through the magnetic field in the $+x$ direction without changing direction?

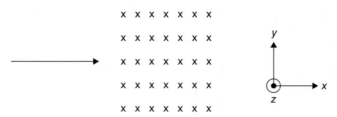

(A) The electric field would be directed in the $+x$ direction.
(B) The electric field would be directied in the $+y$ direction.
(C) The electric field would be directed in the $-y$ direction.
(D) The electric field would be directed in the $+z$ direction.

412. In the illustration, an electron moves into a region with a uniform magnetic field directed out of the page. In what direction would an electric field be added to the magnetic region so that the electron moves in a straight line across the region from left to right?

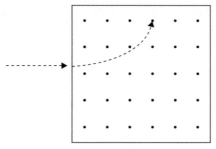

(A) The electric field would be directed into the page.
(B) The electric field would be directed toward the top of the page.
(C) The electric field would be directed toward the bottom of the page.
(D) The electric field would be directed out of the page.

413. In the illustration, an electron enters a magnetic field from the right. Which of the following statements best describes the path of the electron as it travels through the field?

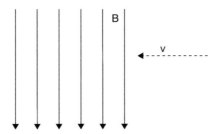

(A) It travels straight through the field undisturbed.
(B) It travels in a circle starting out of the page.
(C) It travels in the direction to which the magnetic field points.
(D) It travels in a circle starting into the page.

414. The illustration shows a beam of protons entering a magnetic field at angle x. Which of the following expressions can be used to determine the magnitude of the magnetic force on each proton as the beam enters the magnetic field?

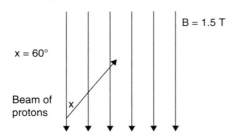

(A) $e(v \cos 60°)B$
(B) $e(v \sin 60°)B$
(C) evB
(D) The magnetic force would be zero.

415. In the illustration, a cathode ray tube is set up between the magnetic poles of a horseshoe magnet. The tube shoots electrons from left to right between the poles. Which of the following statements describes the path of the beam of electrons?

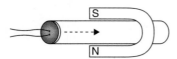

(A) The electrons will curve upward toward the north pole as they reach the region between the poles.
(B) The electrons will curve downward toward the south pole as they reach the region between the poles.
(C) The electrons will maintain a straight path at constant speed through the region between the poles.
(D) The electrons will not move closer to either pole but will curve toward the open end of the magnet and away from the magnet.

416. In the illustration, a very long copper wire is positioned so that it lies between the poles of a strong horseshoe magnet. What is the effect of the magnet on the electrons in the metal wire?

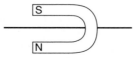

(A) The electrons begin to move to the right.
(B) The electrons begin to move to the left.
(C) The electrons begin to curve to one side of the wire.
(D) The magnet does not affect the electrons in the wire.

417. A charged particle moves into a region with a uniform magnetic field and is observed to move in a circular path in the field. A second charged particle is sent into the field in the same direction but at twice the speed. What difference in the particle's path will be observed?

(A) There will be no difference in the paths of the two particles.
(B) The second particle will move in a circle with a smaller radius.
(C) The second particle will move in a circle with a larger radius.
(D) The second particle will not move in a circular path in the magnetic field.

Forces on Current-Carrying Wires

418. In the illustration, two parallel wires that are a distance d apart have currents of equal magnitude moving in opposite directions. What is the nature of the forces between them?

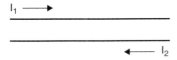

(A) Magnetic forces cause the wires to attract and move toward each other.
(B) Magnetic forces cause the wires to repel and move away from each other.
(C) Electric forces cause the wires to attract and move toward each other.
(D) Electric forces cause the wires to repel and move away from each other.

419. In the illustration, a straight wire carrying a current of 0.5 A runs through a magnetic field of strength 1.5 T. The length of wire in the field is 0.1 m. Determine the magnitude and direction of the force that the magnetic field exerts on the wire.

B = 1.5 T
x x x x x x x
x x x x x x x   I = 0.5 A
───────────────────────
x x x x x x x
x x x x x x x
x x x x x x x
L = 0.1 m

(A) 75 N downward on the page
(B) 7.5 N upward on the page
(C) 0.075 N downward on the page
(D) 0.075 N upward on the page

Electromagnetic Induction

420. In the illustration, the magnetic field is increasing out of the page in the circular wire loop. What current is induced in the loop?

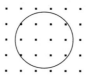

    (A) clockwise
    (B) counterclockwise
    (C) alternating in direction
    (D) No current is induced.

421. In the illustration, a magnet is dropped through a wire loop. Which of the following statements explains what happens in the loop as the magnet enters the plane of the loop and as the magnet continues to drop through and below the loop.

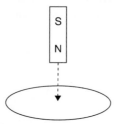

    (A) The current in the loop is counterclockwise (looking downward) the entire time.
    (B) The current in the loop is clockwise (looking downward) the entire time.
    (C) The current in the loop is first clockwise and then counterclockwise.
    (D) The current in the loop is first counterclockwise and then clockwise.

422. In the illustration, a conducting wire loop moves at a constant velocity v into a uniform magnetic field directed into the page. What happens at the instant the loop is halfway into the field?

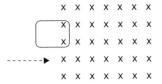

(A) A clockwise current is induced in the loop.
(B) A counterclockwise current is induced in the loop.
(C) A current is induced in the wire only in the part of the loop that is inside the field.
(D) No current is induced in the loop.

423. In the illustration, a hollow coil of coated wire is connected to a galvanometer that measures small electric currents. A strong magnet moves to the left into the coil and through the coil, then exits the coil on the left. What would be the readings on the galvanometer?

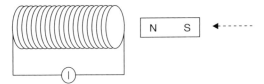

(A) The galvanometer would register a current in one direction as the magnet enters the coil and then read zero as the magnet moves through and exits the coil.
(B) The galvanometer would register a current in one direction the entire time, as the magnet enters the coil, moves through the coil, and exits the coil—decreasing to zero as the magnet moves far away.
(C) The galvanometer would register a current in one direction as the magnet enters the coil and register a current in the opposite direction as the magnet leaves the coil.
(D) No current would be produced in the coil.

424. In the illustration, a conducting wire loop moves at a constant velocity v out of a uniform magnetic field directed into the page. What happens at the instant the loop is halfway out of the field?

```
x  x  x  x  x  x  x

x  x  x  x  x ⌜x  x⌝
                      - - - - - - -▶
x  x  x  x  x ⌞x  x⌟

x  x  x  x  x  x  x

x  x  x  x  x  x  x
```

(A) A clockwise current is induced in the loop.
(B) A counterclockwise current is induced in the loop.
(C) A current is induced in the wire only in the part of the loop that is inside the field.
(D) No current is induced in the loop.

425. A circular loop of wire is rotated through a magnetic field so that the emf induced in the loop fluctuates as a sinusoidal function. The area of the loop is 0.25 m², the strength of the magnetic field is 80 T, and the loop rotates at a rate of 10 Hz. What is the maximum emf induced in the loop?

(A) 5 V
(B) 20 V
(C) 200 V
(D) 800 V

426. In the illustration, the smaller air-core solenoid (coil of wire) on the left is inserted into the larger air-core solenoid on the right without allowing any of the connecting wires to touch. The larger solenoid is connected to a battery, but the smaller solenoid is connected only to an ammeter to read the current in the smaller solenoid. After the smaller solenoid is inside the larger one, the current is turned on. What is observed on the ammeter?

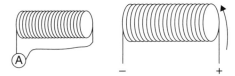

(A) The ammeter will not have a reading, because the smaller solenoid is not connected to a power supply.

(B) The ammeter will have a reading as long as the power is turned on to the larger solenoid, since current is induced in the smaller solenoid by the magnetic field of the larger solenoid.

(C) The ammeter will not have a reading, because the axis of the smaller solenoid is in the same direction as the axis of the larger solenoid.

(D) The ammeter will have a reading as the power is turned on, but the reading will quickly drop to zero again.

427. In the illustration, the smaller air-core solenoid (coil of wire) on the left is inserted into the larger air-core solenoid on the right without allowing any of the connecting wires to touch. The larger solenoid is connected to a battery, but the smaller solenoid is connected only to an ammeter to read the current in the smaller solenoid. After the smaller solenoid is inside the larger one, the current is turned on. There is a quick reading on the ammeter, but the reading goes to zero. To maintain a reading on the ammeter, which of the following actions would be effective?

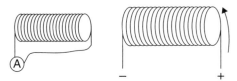

(A) Reconnect the larger solenoid to an alternating current (AC) power supply.

(B) Move both solenoids to the right and keep them moving to the right at the same speed.

(C) Replace the smaller solenoid with a solenoid of the same diameter but with twice as many wire turns.

(D) Place an iron core inside the smaller solenoid.

CHAPTER 13

Light and Optics

Properties of Electromagnetic Radiation

428. Which of the following statements is NOT true regarding electromagnetic waves?

(A) They all travel at the same speed in a vacuum.
(B) They can be polarized.
(C) Frequency is directly proportional to wavelength.
(D) They are formed from oscillating electric and magnetic fields.

429. Which of the following correctly ranks radiations from lowest frequency to highest frequency?

(A) Red, green, infrared, gamma
(B) Infrared, blue, ultraviolet, X-ray
(C) Yellow, red, infrared, radio
(D) Ultraviolet, green, red, infrared

430. Which of the following wavelength ranges falls within the range of ultraviolet light?

(A) 530–600 nm
(B) 250–300 nm
(C) 450–550 nm
(D) 600–700 nm

Interference and Diffraction

431. Interference of light as it passes through a double slit produces a pattern of light and dark bands. Interference is evidence of what property of light?

(A) Light has a particle nature, such that the momentum of photons causes them to cancel their motions when they collide.

(B) Light is attenuated, or absorbed, by the region around the double slits, leaving only certain beams of light and producing a pattern of light and dark.

(C) Light has a wave nature, so that it cannot pass efficiently through the double slits, leaving only certain rays of light to produce a pattern on a screen.

(D) Light has a wave nature, so that the wave patterns produced by the two slits interfere constructively and destructively to produce a pattern.

432. An interference pattern is produced by light from a monochromatic source passing through a double slit. The amplitude of the pattern at the very center is a maximum because the path length difference from each slit to the center of the screen is

(A) zero

(B) maximum

(C) one wavelength

(D) one half wavelength

433. A thin film with an index of refraction of 1.3 is layered on top of glass, so that there is air above the film and glass below the film. In order for green light to be reflected from the film so that the film appears green in full sunlight, the minimum thickness of the film must be

(A) one half the wavelength of green light in air

(B) one fourth the wavelength of green light in the film

(C) one half the wavelength of green light in the film

(D) one fourth the wavelength of green light in air

434. When a large soap bubble is viewed in white light, it produces many colors. Which of the following statements best explains this phenomenon?

(A) Different thicknesses in the bubble reflect different colors.

(B) The bubble acts as a prism and separates the light into a spectrum of colors.

(C) White light is made up of all the colors of the rainbow.

(D) You can view it from any angle, so you see all the colors.

435. As a wave passes through an opening that is approximately equal to its wavelength, the wave will bend or change direction, leading to interference of waves from each side of the opening. This is a demonstration of

(A) diffraction
(B) reflection
(C) refraction
(D) dispersion

436. Using the equation $m\lambda = d \sin \theta$, which of the following conditions is NOT included for fringes produced by single-slit diffraction?

(A) the central maximum of double width
(B) The width of the single slit is d.
(C) Bright fringes occur at $m = 1, 2, 3$, etc.
(D) Dark fringes occur at $m = 1, 2, 3$, etc.

437. As the wavelength of light shining through a single-slit aperture increases, what happens to the interference pattern formed?

(A) Nothing changes in the pattern.
(B) The pattern becomes more spread out.
(C) The pattern moves closer together.
(D) Single slits don't produce interference patterns.

438. In a classroom demonstration, a red laser is shone through a diffraction grating, producing a pattern of bright spots on the wall. Maintaining all other conditions, the red laser is replaced with a green laser. The pattern of bright spots will

(A) move closer together
(B) move farther apart
(C) remain the same, but the central maximum will be much wider
(D) remain the same, but the entire pattern will shift to either the right or left

439. In a diffraction experiment performed on a scale where the slit width is fairly large, the angle θ between bright lines for any set of bright lines becomes very small. In this situation, the diffraction equation, $m\lambda = d \sin \theta$, can take on a simpler form. What is that form, and what is the reason it can be simplified?

(A) $\theta = \dfrac{m\lambda}{d}$, because $\sin \theta$ is almost equal to θ for very small angles.

(B) $\theta = \dfrac{md}{\lambda}$, because the ratio of d to λ is very close to 1.

(C) $\tan \theta = \dfrac{m\lambda}{d}$, because sin and tan are almost equal for very small angles.

(D) $\sin \theta = \dfrac{\lambda}{d}$, because when the angle is small, the functions are the same for all values of m.

Polarization of Light and Doppler Effect

440. Which of the following waves cannot be polarized?
(A) visible light passing through a vacuum
(B) radio waves passing through air
(C) gamma rays passing through a vacuum
(D) sound waves passing through air

441. Which of the following statements is true regarding polarization of light?
(A) The intensity of polarized light is not changed when it passes through a polarizer.
(B) The amount that the intensity of unpolarized light is reduced depends on the incident angle as it reaches the polarizer.
(C) The intensity of polarized light is reduced by half when it passes through a polarizer.
(D) The intensity of polarized light is not affected by the incident angle as it reaches a polarizer.

442. Which of the following statements best describes polarization of light by reflection?

(A) Light reflected from metallic surfaces is usually polarized.

(B) Light reflected from a horizontal surface is generally polarized in the vertical direction.

(C) Reflected light is completely polarized when the reflected beam is perpendicular to the refracted beam.

(D) Polarization is most complete when the light is incident to the surface along the normal.

443. What is the "red shift" of distant objects in the universe?

(A) an observed increase in frequency of light emitted by objects moving away from Earth

(B) an observed decrease in frequency of light emitted by objects moving away from Earth

(C) an observed increase in frequency of light emitted by objects moving toward Earth

(D) an observed decrease in frequency of light emitted by objects moving toward Earth

Reflection, Total Internal Reflection, and Mirrors

444. For total internal reflection to occur at the interface between two different materials, all of the following conditions must be met EXCEPT

(A) the incident path of the light must be from a medium with a higher index of refraction to a medium with a lower index of refraction

(B) the incident angle must be less than the critical angle

(C) the incident angle must be the critical angle when the refracted angle is 90°

(D) the critical angle must be equal to arcsin n_2/n_1, where n_1 is the incident medium

445. The image in a plane mirror of a person standing at a distance d in front of the mirror appears to the person to be

(A) upright, real, and a distance d away

(B) upright, virtual, and a distance $2d$ away

(C) vertically inverted, virtual, and a distance $2d$ from the mirror

(D) vertically inverted, real, and a distance $2d$ from the person

446. In the illustration, four rays from the top of an object strike a mirror and reflect. Each ray and its reflection is shown using a different style of line. Which ray construction does NOT lead to a correct location of the image for the converging mirror shown?

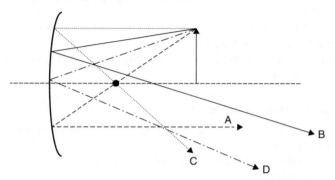

(A) A
(B) B
(C) C
(D) D

447. As a ray of light moves from a medium with a lower index of refraction into a medium with a higher index of refraction,

(A) speed decreases, while frequency and wavelength remain the same
(B) speed and wavelength decrease, while frequency remains the same
(C) speed and wavelength increase, while frequency remains the same
(D) speed and frequency decrease, while wavelength remains the same

448. Which of the following scenarios is NOT possible?

(A) A concave mirror produces a real image.
(B) A plane mirror produces a virtual image.
(C) A convex mirror produces a virtual image.
(D) A concave lens produces a real image.

449. An object placed a distance d_o in front of a convex mirror with a focal length $-f$ produces an image that is one half the size of the original object. Which of the following correctly expresses the focal length?

(A) $-\frac{1}{2}d_o$
(B) $-2d_o$
(C) $-\frac{1}{3}d_o$
(D) $-\frac{1}{4}d_o$

Refraction and Lenses

450. White light entering a glass prism may be separated into its component colors—a phenomenon called *dispersion*—because

(A) each color undergoes a different frequency change as the light goes from the prism back into air
(B) each color has a different index of refraction in the glass
(C) longer wavelengths are refracted more than shorter wavelengths, separating the colors
(D) the red end of the spectrum refracts at a larger angle than the violet

451. Light travels from a medium with an index of refraction n_1 to a medium with an index of refraction n_2, which is greater than n_1. Which of the following must be true for total internal reflection to occur at this interface?

(A) The incident angle must be greater than $45°$.
(B) The incident angle must be less than $45°$.
(C) The incident angle must be greater than arcsin n_2/n_1.
(D) Total internal reflection is not possible in this situation.

452. An object is placed at the focal point of a thin convex lens. Which of the following statements best describes the image that forms?

(A) The image is real, forming at the focal length on the side of the lens opposite the object.
(B) The image is virtual, forming at twice the focal length on the same side of the lens as the object.
(C) The image is real, forming at twice the focal length on the side of the lens opposite the object.
(D) No image will form.

453. A thin diverging lens has a virtual focal length of 12 cm. An object is placed 6 cm from the center of the lens. Which of the following are properties of the image?

(A) real, inverted, 4 cm from the lens
(B) virtual, upright, 6 cm from the lens
(C) virtual, upright, 4 cm from the lens
(D) real, inverted, 6 cm from the lens

454. In the illustration, an object at the position of the arrow is 1.5*f* from the center of a thin convex lens, where *f* is the focal length. Where will the image form?

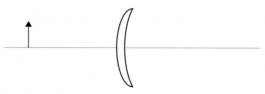

(A) at a distance *f* to the right of the lens
(B) at a distance *f* to the left of the lens
(C) at a distance 2*f* to the right of the lens
(D) at a distance 3*f* to the right of the lens

455. If an optical medium has an average index of refraction of 1.5 for white light, it can be concluded that a ray of white light traveling into the medium

(A) has two thirds the frequency it would have in a vacuum
(B) has two thirds the speed it would have in a vacuum
(C) must change its direction
(D) has 1.5 times the wavelength it would have in a vacuum

456. The thin concave lens in the illustration has a virtual focal length *f*. An object, represented by the arrow, is positioned at a distance 1.5*f* from the center of the lens. Where will the image form?

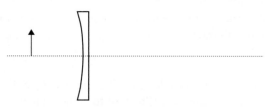

(A) at a distance 3*f* to the right of the lens
(B) at a distance 3*f* to the left of the lens
(C) at a distance 3*f*/5 to the left of the lens
(D) at a distance 3*f*/5 to the right of the lens

457. An object that looks blue when viewed under a white light source will appear to be which color when illuminated by white light and viewed through a yellow filter?

(A) orange
(B) black
(C) red
(D) green

458. When white light travels from air into a glass prism and is dispersed into colors,

(A) blue light refracts over a smaller angle than red
(B) all frequencies of light travel at the same speed
(C) green light changes wavelength more than blue
(D) blue light has a lower speed than red

459. One lens with a focal length of 0.5 m and a second lens with a focal length of 0.25 m are brought into close contact. What is the lens strength, in diopters, of the combination of the two lenses?

(A) 2
(B) 4
(C) 6
(D) 8

460. One lens with a strength of 1.25 diopters and a second lens with a strength of 2 diopters are brought into contact. What is the approximate focal length of the combination of the two lenses?

(A) 5 cm
(B) 8 cm
(C) 24 cm
(D) 33 cm

461. Which of the following statements provides the cause of and a possible solution for spherical lens aberration?

(A) Spherical aberration is produced when a lens is not perfectly spherical, causing light to focus at multiple points. Both sides of the lens should be ground so that it is perfectly spherical.

(B) Spherical aberration is produced when a lens bends different wavelengths of light by different amounts, causing multiple focal points. Making the lens more spherical will cause red light to bend more, reducing the effect.

(C) Spherical aberration is produced when the lens is ground so the focal length is greater than $R/2$, where R is the radius of curvature. Grinding the lens so that it is spherical but has less curvature will improve focus.

(D) Spherical aberration is produced when a spherical lens bends light from the edges to a closer focal point than light passing through closer to the center. Making the lens nonspherical will improve focus.

462. Which of the following statements describes the eye of a myopic (nearsighted) person and a possible solution?

(A) In nearsightedness, light passing through the eye's lens is focused in front of the retina, that is, the focal length of the lens is less than the distance from the lens to the retina. A convex lens will increase the focal length to correct it.

(B) In nearsightedness, light passing through the eye's lens is focused behind the retina, that is, the focal length of the lens is more than the distance from the lens to the retina. A convex lens will increase the focal length to correct it.

(C) In nearsightedness, light passing through the eye's lens is focused behind the retina, that is, the focal length of the lens is more than the distance from the lens to the retina. A concave lens will decrease the focal length to correct it.

(D) In nearsightedness, light passing through the eye's lens is focused in front of the retina, that is, the focal length of the lens is less than the distance from the lens to the retina. A concave lens will increase the focal length to correct it.

463. A biology student inspects a slide by using a microscope that has a 5× eyepiece lens and by setting the objective lens at 10×. An object on the slide that is 0.3 mm in diameter will appear to have what diameter?

(A) 0.15 cm

(B) 0.45 cm

(C) 1.5 cm

(D) 4.5 cm

464. A student is making a refracting telescope from two lenses. First, the student tests each lens and determines that the objective lens focuses light from distant objects at a point 15 cm from the lens. The eyepiece lens focuses light from distant objects at a point 5 cm from the lens. When constructing the telescope, the lenses need to be placed at each end of a tube that is how long?

(A) 75 cm
(B) 40 cm
(C) 20 cm
(D) 3 m

Lasers

465. Laser light must be both

(A) monochromatic and coherent
(B) polarized and monochromatic
(C) polarized and coherent
(D) monochromatic and diffuse

466. Which of the following statements must be true for production of laser light?

(A) Electrons in the atom are stimulated to a higher energy state and then move back to the ground state, emitting visible light.
(B) Electrons in a metastable state emit photons of higher energy than the ground state.
(C) A population inversion of electrons exists between the metastable state within the atoms.
(D) Photons excite electrons to a metastable state corresponding to the energy of the ground state.

CHAPTER 14

Atomic and Nuclear Physics

Emission Spectrum of Hydrogen (Bohr Model)

467. The energy diagram shows the first four energy states and possible transitions for an electron in an atom. Which transition would emit a photon with the highest frequency?

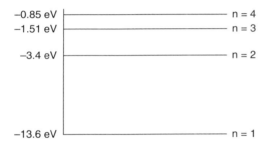

(A) $n = 4$ to $n = 2$
(B) $n = 1$ to $n = 3$
(C) $n = 3$ to $n = 1$
(D) $n = 1$ to $n = 4$

468. In the Bohr model of the atom, if the energy of an electron in the lowest energy state (ground state) is E, what is the energy of an electron in energy n?

(A) nE
(B) E/n
(C) n^2E
(D) E/n^2

469. In the Bohr model of the atom, if R is the orbital radius of an electron in the lowest energy state, what would the orbital radius of an electron in the third energy level be?

(A) $2R$
(B) $3R$
(C) $6R$
(D) $9R$

470. Which of the following statements is true regarding the development of the Bohr model of the atom?

(A) Compared to the previous Rutherford model, the Bohr model emphasized the structure of the nucleus.
(B) The Bohr model was a planetary model for the electron, with the electron orbiting the nucleus in a circular path around the nucleus.
(C) The Bohr model had electrons orbiting at only certain distances from the nucleus, corresponding to specific energies.
(D) All of the above

Quantized Energy States for Electrons

471. In the Bohr model of the hydrogen atom, the electron is confined to specific energy states. If n is the quantum number for a particular energy level, λ_n is the electron wavelength associated with that energy level, and R is the radius for the specified energy level, then which of the following equations must be correct?

(A) $2\pi R = n\lambda$
(B) $2\pi\lambda = nR$
(C) $\pi R = n\lambda$
(D) $R^2 = n\lambda$

472. Determine the wavelength for an electron in the Bohr model of the hydrogen atom, if the electron is in energy state $n = 1$ with an energy E.

(A) $\lambda = \dfrac{hc}{E}$

(B) $\lambda = \dfrac{E}{h}$

(C) $\lambda = \dfrac{h}{E}$

(D) $\lambda = \dfrac{hf}{E}$

Refer to the energy diagram for questions 473 and 474.

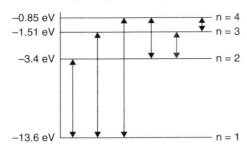

473. The energy diagram shows the absorption/emission spectrum for hydrogen. What is the smallest energy possible for an emitted photon from hydrogen?

(A) 13.6 eV
(B) 3.4 eV
(C) 0.85 eV
(D) 0.66 eV

474. The energy diagram shows the absorption/emission spectrum for hydrogen. What energy transition would emit a photon with the shortest wavelength?

(A) $n = 2$ to $n = 1$
(B) $n = 3$ to $n = 2$
(C) $n = 4$ to $n = 1$
(D) $n = 4$ to $n = 3$

Energy of Photo Emission and Absorption

475. An electron changes energy states from higher energy E_2 to lower energy E_1. Which of the following correctly expresses the wavelength of light emitted in this transition?

(A) $\dfrac{hf}{E_2 - E_1}$

(B) $\dfrac{hc}{E_2 - E_1}$

(C) $\dfrac{f}{E_2 - E_1}$

(D) $\dfrac{E_2 - E_1}{hc}$

476. The graph represents data from a photoelectric effect experiment. Estimate the minimum (cutoff) frequency of light that will cause ejection of electrons from zinc.

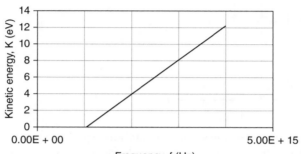

(A) 5.0×10^{14} Hz
(B) 2.5×10^{15} Hz
(C) 2.0×10^{15} Hz
(D) 1.0×10^{15} Hz

Atomic Number and Atomic Weight

477. What does the symbol $^4_2$He for the element helium mean?

(A) An atom of helium has 2 protons and 4 electrons.
(B) A helium nucleus has 2 protons and 4 neutrons.
(C) A helium nucleus has 2 protons and 2 neutrons.
(D) An atom of helium has 2 protons and a total of 4 charged nucleons.

478. Which of the following statements is NOT true regarding atomic nuclei?

(A) All atomic nucleons are protons and neutrons.
(B) All atomic nuclei have an approximately constant density, regardless of composition.
(C) All nuclei of a given element have the same number of protons.
(D) All nuclei of a given element have the same total number of nucleons.

Neutrons, Protons, and Isotopes

479. Which of the following is a fundamental particle?

(A) proton
(B) neutron
(C) electron
(D) deuteron

480. Which of the following is NOT an isotope of hydrogen?

(A) protium

(B) deuterium

(C) tritium

(D) quaternium

481. Which of the following nuclear transformations is NOT possible?

(A) decay of a neutron into a proton and an electron

(B) capture of an electron by a proton to produce a neutron

(C) emission of a positron by a proton to produce a neutron

(D) decay of a proton into a neutron and an electron

482. What is the general pattern for the number of neutrons in stable isotopes?

(A) The most stable isotopes always have an equal number of protons and neutrons in the nucleus.

(B) The ratio of neutrons to protons tends to increase in stable isotopes as atomic number increases.

(C) The ratio of neutrons to protons tends to decrease in stable isotopes as atomic number increases.

(D) There seems to be no general pattern for the ratio of neutrons to protons for stable isotopes as the sizes of nuclei increase.

Weak and Strong Forces

483. What is the weak nuclear force?

(A) the force that loosely binds outer shell electrons to the nucleus of an atom

(B) the force that holds the nucleus together

(C) the force that causes protons in the nucleus to repel each other

(D) the nuclear force responsible for beta decay

484. Which of the following fundamental forces is considered to be the strongest at short ranges?

(A) gravitational force

(B) the weak nuclear force

(C) the strong nuclear force

(D) electromagnetic force

Radioactive Decay

485. As a result of the emission of an alpha particle, an atomic nucleus

(A) increases its atomic number by 2 and increases its mass number by 4
(B) decreases its atomic number by 2 and decreases its mass number by 4
(C) increases its atomic number by 2 and decreases its mass number by 4
(D) decreases its atomic number by 2 and increases its mass number by 4

486. As a result of the emission of a beta particle, an atomic nucleus

(A) increases its atomic number by 2 and increases its mass number by 1
(B) increases its atomic number by 1 but doesn't change its mass number
(C) increases its atomic number by 1 and decreases its mass number by 1
(D) decreases its atomic number by 1 and increases its mass number by 1

487. During radioactive emission of gamma radiation in which no other particles are emitted, the gamma photons are emitted in pairs. Which conservation law would be defied if only one gamma photon were emitted?

(A) conservation of mass
(B) conservation of charge
(C) conservation of linear momentum
(D) conservation of energy

488. The radioactive element radium-224 has a half-life of 3.66 days. Which of the following statements is true regarding one nucleus of radium after 3.66 days?

(A) Half of the nucleus has decayed.
(B) The nucleus will decay only when a second nucleus is brought into contact with it.
(C) There is a 50% chance the nucleus will have decayed.
(D) The nucleus won't decay prior to 3.66 days, but should decay after that time.

489. What nuclear transformation occurs during beta decay?

(A) A proton decays into a neutron and an electron.
(B) An electron and proton combine to form a neutron.
(C) A neutron decays into a proton and an electron.
(D) An electron and a neutron combine to form a proton.

490. The chart shows the decay curve for a 100 g sample of polonium-210. Which of the following best estimates the half-life of ^{210}Po?

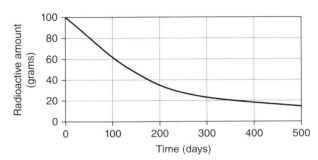

(A)   500 days
(B)   250 days
(C)   180 days
(D)   140 days

491. Particles with mass may be given off by a nucleus through the process of radioactive decay, thus reducing the mass of the nucleus. Which of the following is NOT one of these particles?

(A)   gammas
(B)   positrons
(C)   electrons
(D)   alpha particles

492. One step in the radioactive decay series of uranium-235 to lead-207 is the decay of bismuth-215. In this step, what is produced when $^{215}_{83}$Bi gives off an alpha particle and a beta particle?

(A) $^{218}_{85}$At
(B) $^{211}_{82}$Pb
(C) $^{211}_{83}$Bi
(D) $^{211}_{84}$Po

493. A radioactive sample is placed in a cloud chamber so that the paths of radioactive decay products can be seen as "tracks" in the chamber. A magnetic field is set up across the cloud chamber to help identify the decay products. Which of the following radioactive decay products would never change direction in the magnetic field?

(A) alpha particles
(B) beta particles
(C) gamma rays
(D) positrons

Fission and Fusion

494. In the nuclear fission reaction

$$^{235}_{92}U + {}^{1}_{0}n \rightarrow {}^{139}_{56}Ba + {}^{94}_{36}Kr + \underline{\qquad}$$

a uranium atom is bombarded with a neutron to produce an atom of barium and an atom of krypton. What is the other product of this reaction?

(A) an electron
(B) two electrons
(C) a proton
(D) three neutrons

495. In a nuclear fusion reaction, four protons (hydrogen nuclei) combine to form a helium nucleus, two neutrinos, and another product.

$$4^{1}_{1}H \rightarrow {}^{4}_{2}He + 2^{0}_{0}\eta + \underline{\qquad}$$

What is the other product of this reaction?

(A) a helium nucleus
(B) two protons
(C) two positrons (positive electrons)
(D) two beta particles (negative electrons)

496. According to some scientists, the fusion of deuterium with tritium to create helium-4 may be a source of energy in the future, since the reaction gives off large amounts of energy.

$$^{2}_{1}H + {}^{3}_{1}H \rightarrow {}^{4}_{2}He + \underline{\qquad} + energy$$

What is the other product of this reaction?

(A) a proton
(B) a neutron
(C) an electron
(D) a positron

Mass-Energy Equivalence

497. Which of the following equations correctly expresses the momentum of a photon?

(A) $p = \dfrac{hf}{c}$

(B) $p = \dfrac{h}{c}$

(C) $p = hf$

(D) $p = h\lambda$

498. The number 931 MeV/c² is a measurement of a particle's

(A) momentum

(B) mass

(C) energy

(D) velocity

499. When a nucleus in an excited state emits a gamma photon,

(A) a neutron in the nucleus is converted to a proton of higher energy

(B) the reduction in mass of the nucleus corresponds to the energy of the gamma photon

(C) the mass number of the nucleus is reduced, accounting for the energy of the emitted photon

(D) the atomic number is reduced, accounting for the energy of the emitted photon

500. Under certain conditions, a particle-antiparticle pair (such as an electron and a positron) can annihilate each other, converting all the mass of the particles into two gamma photons. If m is the mass of each particle, which of the following equations can be used to determine the frequency of each photon?

(A) $f = \dfrac{2mc^2}{\lambda}$

(B) $f = \dfrac{mc^2}{2h}$

(C) $f = \dfrac{mc^2}{h}$

(D) $f = \dfrac{2mc^2}{h}$

ANSWERS

Note: In this book, either $g = 9.8$ m/s^2 or $g = 10$ m/s^2 may be used in solutions that involve calculations. Since the answers are rounded, either value will provide the correct answer.

Chapter 1: Kinematics: Motion in One and Two Dimensions

1. (C) The units on the left side of the equation are (m/s)^2, or m^2/s^2. On the right, the units on acceleration are m/s^2 and units on displacement are m; thus the units on the right side are (m/s^2)(m), or m^2/s^2. The correct answer is also recognizable from the familiar equation $v_f^2 = v_o^2 + 2as$ for the case where v_o^2 is equal to zero.

2. (B) Graph II shows a power curve, or the relationship "y as a function of x^2." Graph I might represent the shape of an inverse curve, or the relationship "y as a function of $1/x$." Graph III might represent the shape of a root curve, or the relationship "y as a function of square root of x." Choice (D) is a distractor—it is not a good representation of a mathematical curve (perhaps coming closest to a decreasing exponential function or a graph of a circle centered on (0,0) with x and y both positive).

3. (A) Analysis of units can be an important tool in determining the meanings of slope and area in situations where there is some difficulty in understanding the meanings of these quantities. Slope is "rise over run," or y axis quantity divided by x axis quantity. In this case, the slope is newtons per meter (N/m), which might be the spring constant, for example, if the graph is Spring Force as a Function of Spring Extension. The area under the graph has units determined by multiplying the units on the axes. In this case, the units are newton·meters (N·m), which would be the work done in stretching a spring a given distance for the example described.

4. (B) First, convert centimeters to meters; this needs to be done in every case where you must determine work or energy in joules when using newtons for force. One meter is equivalent to 100 cm, so the decimal is moved two places to the left in each case to convert cm to m. In choice (A), force times distance is (5)(2), or 10 J. In choice (B), force times distance is (5)(0.2), or 1.0 J—the correct answer. In choice (C), force times distance is (50)(.002) or (50)(2)/1000, which is 0.1 J. In choice (D), force times distance is (5)(0.02), or 0.1 J.

5. (C) The prefix *micro-* means one millionth, or 1×10^{-6}, while the prefix *mega-* means one million, or 1×10^6. One meter is equivalent to one million micrometers, and one megameter is equivalent to one million meters. Therefore, one megameter is equivalent to one million times one million micrometers, or one trillion (1×10^{12}) micrometers. The unit cancellation method can also be used to convert units.

$$\frac{(1 \times 10^6 \text{ μm})}{1 \text{ m}} \times \frac{(1 \times 10^6 \text{ m})}{1 \text{ Mm}} = \frac{(1 \times 10^{12} \text{ μm})}{1 \text{ Mm}}$$

Each fraction multiplied is an "equivalent," where the numerator and denominator are equal, so this essentially involves multiplying by one in each case. Units are canceled in the numerator and denominator to determine the answer.

6. (A) The units in choice (A) are obtained by multiplying the quantities as shown, making sure to square the units on Y, and canceling one meter in the numerator with the meter in the denominator. In fact, the formula in choice (A) is equivalent to one newton $(1 \text{ kg·m/s}^2.)$ This formula is also a method of calculating centripetal force on an object of mass m (in kg) moving at speed v (in m/s) in a circle of radius R (in meters). The force is the result, measured in newtons.

7. (D) From the choices, it's obvious that we need to substitute for the newton (1 kg·m/s^2). Substituting this for the quantity X, substituting kg·m for the quantity Y, and canceling yield the square root of meters squared per seconds squared, which produces m/s.

$$\sqrt{\frac{\left(\dfrac{\text{kg·m}}{s^2}\right)}{\left(\dfrac{\text{kg}}{m}\right)}} = \sqrt{\left(\frac{\text{kg·m}}{s^2}\right)\left(\frac{m}{\text{kg}}\right)} = \sqrt{\frac{m^2}{s^2}} = \text{m/s}$$

This is a real determination for the speed of a wave on a string, where X represents the tension in the string (in newtons) and Y represents the linear density of the string (in kg/m). The speed, indeed, is measured in meters per second.

8. (A) If the quantities n, R, and T are constant in the equation $PV = nRT$, then the product PV is equal to a constant. P and V are therefore inversely proportional to each other. Graph I represents an inverse proportion of the form $xy = $ constant, so this is the correct choice. Graph II represents the form $y = kx^2$, where k is a constant. Graph III represents the form $y = k\sqrt{x}$, where k is a constant. Graph IV is a distractor (perhaps coming closest to a decreasing exponential function or a graph of a circle centered on $(0,0)$ with x and y both positive).

9. (C) If length is the independent variable and period is the dependent variable, then the equation is of the form "period is a function of length." Period would be plotted on the y axis and length would be plotted on the x axis, and the graph would be of the form $y = k\sqrt{x}$, shown in Graph III. Graph I represents an inverse proportion of the form $xy = $ constant, so this is an incorrect choice. Graph II represents the form $y = kx^2$, where k is a constant. Graph IV is a distractor (perhaps coming closest to a decreasing exponential function or a graph of a circle centered on $(0,0)$ with x and y both positive).

10. (B) The graph is of the form $y = kx^2$, so squaring all the values of X in the data and plotting "Y as a function of X^2" should produce a linear graph. A linear graph can also be produced by plotting "Y^2 as a function of X."

11. (A) Vectors are added from tip to tail, with the resultant, or sum, measured from the beginning of the first vector to the end of the second, as shown by the dashed line from the start of vector X to the end of vector Y.

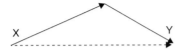

12. (B) The airplane's displacement is expressed in terms of components north of A and east of A. The first portion of the flight is 300 km north with no component east. The second portion of the flight is expressed in terms of components of a right triangle with acute angles of 45°. Since this type of triangle has sides with length ratios of 1-1-$\sqrt{2}$, the sides must be 1,000 km, 1,000 km, and 1,400 km (since $\sqrt{2}$ = 1.4). This means that the components for the second portion of the flight are 1,000 km north and 1,000 km east. Adding these values to those of the first portion of the flight, the displacement is 1,300 km north and 1,000 km east. (It's helpful to recognize the length ratios for the sides of special triangles like the one here.)

13. (C) Since the two forces are at right angles, they can be considered to be components of the resultant force; this is recognized as a 3-4-5 right triangle. The net force is 50 N. Newton's second law, $\Sigma F = ma$, is used to determine the acceleration.

$$a = \frac{\Sigma F}{m} = \frac{50 \text{ N}}{35 \text{ kg}} = 1.4 \text{ m/s}^2$$

14. (C) The magnitude of the resultant of two vectors that are perpendicular to each other can be determined using the Pythagorean theorem. Since the question asks only for speed, which is not a vector, the direction of the resultant is not part of the answer.

$$R = \sqrt{A^2 + B^2} = \sqrt{200^2 + 70^2}$$

15. (C) The resultant of vector A minus vector B is the addition of vector A to the negative of vector B. The negative of a vector has the same magnitude, but the vector is in the opposite direction. The addition of vector A to $-$B is shown as a dashed arrow in the illustration.

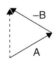

16. (D) The slope of the line is the acceleration, and since the slope is constant, the acceleration is constant. Any two points on the line can be used to determine the slope, which is negative.

$$\text{Slope} = \frac{\Delta y}{\Delta x} = \frac{0 - 6 \text{ m/s}}{6 \text{ m/s} - 0} = -1 \text{ m/s}^2$$

17. (D) Acceleration can be determined by using the equation $x = v_o t + \frac{1}{2}at^2$ for the first interval, with the initial velocity equal to zero: $2\text{ m} = 0 + \frac{1}{2}a(4\text{ s})^2$, yielding an acceleration of $\frac{1}{4}$ m/s². This acceleration is then used to determine the final velocity after that first interval.

$$v_f = v_o + at = 0 + (\frac{1}{4}\text{ m/s}^2)(4\text{ s}) = 1\text{ m/s}$$

Now, the original equation is applied again for the second interval, with the initial velocity 1 m/s, to determine the distance traveled.

$$x = v_o t + \frac{1}{2}at^2 = (1)(4\text{ s}) + \frac{1}{2}(\frac{1}{4})(4\text{ s})^2 = 6\text{ m}$$

There is a shortcut method. An object starting from rest and accelerating at a constant rate will travel distances in equal intervals of time in the ratio of the odd numbers: 1, 3, 5, 7, etc. In this case, the first distance is 2 m, so the distance traveled during the second equal time interval is 3 times 2, or 6 m. (This shortcut method, sometimes called "Galileo's law of odd numbers," is very useful for objects starting from rest under the influence of the gravitational force.)

18. (C) For a graph with velocity on the y axis and time on the x axis, the slope would be $\Delta y / \Delta x$, or $\Delta v / \Delta t$. This ratio would have units of m/s/s, which are units of acceleration. Since only a single point is designated, the slope for this point is the instantaneous acceleration, or acceleration at that instant in time.

19. (D) In choice (A), the acceleration is centripetal and is constant if the motion is at uniform speed. In choice (B), the acceleration could be constant and positive, while in choice (C) the acceleration could be constant and negative. Thus, all could be true, and the correct answer is choice (D).

20. (D) Choice (A), (B), or (C) could be true. If the line is horizontal, the velocity is constant. If the line is diagonal, the slope is the acceleration, which is constant. If the line is a horizontal line at $v = 0$, both velocity and acceleration are zero.

21. (C) A parabolic path is defined by an object in free motion in two dimensions if there is a constant net force on the object in one dimension and no net force in the second dimension. If there is no net force in one of the dimensions, there is no acceleration ($\Sigma F = ma$) and, therefore, constant velocity, while in the other dimension, there would be a constant force, which means constant acceleration in that dimension. An object projected into the air at an angle to the ground will take a parabolic path if frictional effects due to air are disregarded.

22. (D) The area between the graph line and the x axis is the change in position. In this graph, the area is positive and is equal to $(\frac{1}{2})(6\text{ m/s})(6\text{ s})$, since the shape is a triangle. The displacement, then, is 18 m. Further, the area for the time interval from 6 s to 10 s is negative (-8 m), so the total displacement from $t = 0$ to $t = 10$ is 10 m. This graph tells us that the object moved in the positive direction for the first 6 seconds and then in the negative direction for the next 4 seconds.

23. (D) The slope of a tangent line at the time $t = 7$ seconds is the velocity, which in this case is negative. The slope, or "rise over run," can be estimated by approximating the curve as a line from the points (6,10) to (7.4,0). Thus, the closest estimate of the velocity is $-10/1.5$ m/s, which is about -7 m/s.

24. (B) According to this graph, the object starts moving forward from a "zero" position of $x = 10$ at a velocity of about 5 m/s (the slope). The object decreases its velocity from $t = 0$ to $t = 3$, reaching a velocity of zero at $t = 3$ s. The object then turns around at $t = 3$ and increases its velocity in the negative direction from $t = 3$ to $t = 10$ s, reaching a point 30 m behind the "zero" position and 40 m behind the point where it started.

25. (A) The acceleration of the air rocket, due to the gravitational force exerted on it, is downward during the entire trip of the rocket—which is, by our definition, always negative. The velocity vector, which describes the direction of motion of the rocket, is, by our definition, positive while the rocket is on its way upward and negative as it falls back down.

26. (C) Assuming negligible air friction, the ball moves upward during the first 2 s of its motion and downward for the next 2 s. Its vertical motion is independent of its horizontal motion, so it travels upward until the vertical component of its velocity is zero and then falls for 2 s. Therefore, at a time 3 s after it leaves the ground, the ball has moved upward for 2 s and fallen for 1 s.

27. (B) Once the stone leaves the thrower's hand, it is only under the influence of the gravitational force, which produces a downward force and downward acceleration. The acceleration is the same at every moment during the stone's trip upward and back down again, and that constant acceleration is 9.8 m/s².

28. (A) Solve for time, t, in the equation for the vertical motion of the wheel. Since the vertical motion is independent of the horizontal motion, the speed of the wheel horizontally as it falls does not affect the time it takes to drop to the ground.

$$\Delta y = v_{oy}t + \tfrac{1}{2}at^2$$
$$-500 \text{ m} = 0 + \tfrac{1}{2}(-10 \text{ m/s}^2)t^2$$
$$t = 10 \text{ s}$$

29. (D) When the rocket is fired vertically, its vertical velocity is maximum, so the rocket reaches its maximum height. When it is fired at an angle of less than 90°, only the vertical component determines the vertical height, and the vertical component of the velocity decreases as the angle decreases. The rocket's time in the air is determined by its altitude, so the time is maximum when the vertical velocity is maximum. When fired at an angle of 60° to the ground, the vertical velocity component is less than v and air time is less than t.

30. (B) Assuming negligible air friction, the ball reached the top of its path in half the time (2 s). At the peak of its motion, the ball had a velocity of zero, so it fell from rest for the next 2 s, reaching a final velocity at the bottom of its path that is theoretically the same magnitude as the velocity when it started its path upward.

$$v_f = v_o + at = 0 + (10 \text{ m/s}^2)(2 \text{ s}) = 20 \text{ m/s}$$

31. (D) The time it takes the rock to fall to the ground depends only on the height of the building and is independent of the horizontal speed.

$$\Delta y = v_{oy}t + \frac{1}{2}at^2$$
$$-h = 0 + \frac{1}{2}(-g)t^2$$
$$t = \sqrt{\frac{2h}{g}}$$

32. (D) Assuming negligible air friction, horizontal acceleration is zero, but vertical acceleration is a constant value of g downward at every point along the projectile's path. Thus, the acceleration is never zero. The horizontal speed remains constant. Vertical speed is maximum at A, decreases to zero at C, and then increases to a maximum at E just before it lands. The height is maximum at point C.

33. (C) Since the wind vector and the plane vector are at right angles, the resultant vector can be determined using the Pythagorean theorem.

$$v = \sqrt{v_w^2 + v_p^2} = \sqrt{100^2 + 10^2}$$

Even without the final calculation, it is easy to see that the resultant speed is closer to 101 km/h than to 110 km/h. The direction will not be due northeast, since the wind causes the plane to veer east. The resultant direction will be a small angle, since the tangent of the angle is the wind speed divided by the plane's air speed. That small angle is east of north.

34. (C) The boat's resultant path is the sum of the boat's velocity vector (pointing across the river) and the river's velocity vector (pointing to the right). Path 3 is the most logical resultant of these vectors, so the boat will move downstream before reaching the other side of the river. The boat and velocity vectors, 6 m/s and 8 m/s, respectively, are in a ratio of 3:4, so they form the legs of a right triangle. This is one of the special right triangles, a 3-4-5 right triangle, so the resultant velocity vector follows the same ratio. The boat will move downstream at a speed of 10 m/s.

35. (A) Since the block is in parabolic motion from the time it leaves the table until it hits the floor, its acceleration in the vertical direction is g (9.8 m/s^2) and there is no acceleration in the horizontal direction.

36. (C) The horizontal and vertical motions of the block are independent, linked only by time (since both components of motion occur during the same time). The horizontal component of velocity remains constant at 2 m/s during the block's trip to the ground. The vertical velocity increases as the block falls with an acceleration of g. Note that the initial vertical velocity is zero, since the block leaves the roof moving only horizontally. Using $g = 10$ m/s^2, the final vertical velocity is calculated.

$$v_f^2 = v_o^2 + 2as$$
$$v_f^2 = 0 + (2)(10 \text{ m/s}^2)(5 \text{ m}) = 100$$
$$v_f = 10 \text{ m/s}$$

Chapter 2: Forces and Newton's Laws of Motion

37. (D) Find the x and y coordinates of the center of mass separately, using the equations below and the total mass of the three objects (10 g).

$$x_{com} = \frac{m_1 x_1 + m_2 x_2 + m_3 x_3}{m_{total}} = \frac{(2)(0) + (6)(5) + (2)(2)}{10} = 3.4$$

$$y_{com} = \frac{m_1 y_1 + m_2 y_2 + m_3 y_3}{m_{total}} = \frac{(2)(7) + (6)(6) + (2)(2)}{10} = 5.4$$

38. (D) The center of mass can be determined as an average position in each of the x and y coordinate directions. In the x direction, add the three coordinates to get -3 and divide by 3 (since there are 3 items) to get -1. In the y direction, the coordinate is the sum of the three coordinates divided by 3, which is 6/3, or 2. So the center of mass is located at the point $(-1, 2)$. The actual equations are: $x_{com} = \Sigma mx/m_{total}$ and $y_{com} = \Sigma my/m_{total}$. Since the three objects are equal in mass, they cancel, and the coordinates add in the manner shown above.

39. (D) The acceleration of the car is determined by finding the change in velocity and dividing by time. This can be done without a calculator by determining that the change in speed is 40 m/s. Then, change in speed is divided by time, yielding an acceleration of 10 m/s². Finally, Newton's second law of motion is applied, using the mass of the car and the acceleration to determine the magnitude of the force. (Of course, both the acceleration and force are negative, because the velocity of the car is reduced, but the question only asks for the magnitude of the average force.)

$$\vec{a} = \frac{\vec{v}_f - \vec{v}_o}{t} = \frac{30 \text{ m/s} - 70 \text{ m/s}}{4 \text{ s}} = -10 \text{ m/s}^2$$

$$\vec{F} = m\vec{a} = (500 \text{ kg})(-10 \text{ m/s}^2) = -5{,}000 \text{ N}$$

40. (B) The acceleration of an object or system is directly proportional to the net force exerted on the object or system and inversely proportional to its mass.

$$\Sigma F = ma$$

$$a = \frac{\Sigma F}{m}$$

On the plot of Acceleration as a Function of Force, the slope would be $1/m$. Use the data point $(4,10)$ on the line to calculate slope, since the best-fit line goes through that point and through the origin. The slope is $\Delta y/\Delta x$, or 10/6. Since the slope is $1/m$, the mass is 6/10 kg, or 0.6 kg.

41. (C) According to Newton's third law of motion, for every action there is an equal and opposite reaction, with action and reaction forces on separate bodies. In this case, the force of the truck pulling forward on the trailer is equal to the force of the trailer pulling backward on the truck.

42. (D) Newton's second law, $\Sigma F = ma$, is applied. The product ma equals 10 N, so the net force must be 10 N. The (backward) friction force must be 2 N, so the sum of 12 N forward and 2 N backward must be 10 N.

43. (C) Considering the frame of reference where one axis is along the surface of the ramp, the sum of all forces on the box that are parallel to the ramp must equal zero in order for the box to remain stationary. The component of W that points downward along the ramp is $W \sin \theta$. This component must be equal to the two forces directed upward along the ramp, which are the tension T and the friction force F_F.

44. (D) As the ramp angle is increased, the normal force from the ramp decreases. Since friction depends on the coefficient of friction (which doesn't change) and normal force, the friction force decreases as the normal force decreases. As the ramp is tilted, more of the weight of the block is supported by the string, so the tension increases.

45. (A) Newton's second law of motion, $\Sigma F = ma$, is used to solve for tension. To determine the mass of the elevator car, its weight in newtons is divided by g. The mass is 1,000 kg.

$$\Sigma F = T - W = ma$$
$$T = W + ma = 10,000 \text{ N} + (1,000 \text{ kg})(3.0 \text{ m/s}^2) = 13,000 \text{ N}$$

46. (D) Newton's second law of motion, $\Sigma F = ma$, is used to solve for acceleration.

$$a = \frac{\Sigma F}{m} = \frac{10 \text{ N}}{15 \text{ kg}} = 0.67 \text{ m/s}^2$$

47. (D) Newton's second law of motion, $\Sigma F = ma$, is used to solve for change in speed.

$$\Sigma F = m \frac{\Delta v}{\Delta t}$$
$$\Delta v = \frac{\Sigma F(t)}{m} = \frac{(10 \text{ N})(5 \text{ s})}{2 \text{ kg}} = 25 \text{ m/s}$$

Only choice (D) has a change in speed of 25 m/s.

48. (D) The vectors 30 N north and 40 N east are components of the resultant vector that accelerates the object. Consider a 3-4-5 right triangle, where the hypotenuse would be the resultant of 50 N. Then, use Newton's second law of motion to determine the acceleration.

$$a = \frac{\Sigma F}{m} = \frac{50 \text{ N}}{35 \text{ kg}} = 1.4 \text{ m/s}^2$$

49. (B) Consider the three connected blocks as a system with a total mass of 6 kg. Using the equation $a = F/m$, the acceleration is 2 m/s². Since choice (B) or (C) must therefore be correct, the tension in the string attached to the 1 kg block only must accelerate that block, so it must be less than 12 N; there is no need to actually make the calculation. (Using $F = ma$ to determine the tension, 1 kg [the mass] × 2 m/s² [the acceleration] = 2 N [the tension].)

50. (B) When the elevator car is accelerating upward, there are two forces on the person—the gravitational force downward and the normal force of the scale upward. For the person to accelerate upward, there must be more force upward on the person than downward ($\Sigma F = ma$). The scale reading is equal to the weight of the person when in equilibrium—either stationary or moving up or down at constant speed. The scale reading is more than the person's weight when the person is accelerating upward, and the scale reading is less than the person's weight when the person is accelerating downward. The scale would read zero only if the scale and the person were in free fall.

51. (C) The forces on the 200 N frame are vectors and must be considered in each direction separately. In the y direction, the only force downward is 200 N. In the upward direction, each of the two components of tension supports half of that, so the vertical component of each tension is equal to 100 N. Using the 1-1-$\sqrt{2}$ relationship in a right triangle that has 45° angles, we determine that each of the components is 100 N and the tension (the hypotenuse) must be $100\sqrt{2}$, which is 100×1.4, or about 140 N. This choice is also the most reasonable.

52. (B) Newton's second law of motion is applied to solve for acceleration.

$$\Sigma F = ma$$

$$a = \frac{\Sigma F}{m} = \frac{10 \text{ N}}{1 \text{ kg}} = 10 \text{ m/s}^2$$

53. (C) The weight of the rock is the gravitational force of the hypothetical planet on the rock.

$$F_G = \frac{GMm}{R^2}$$

On Earth, the gravitational force is 12 N. If the rock is moved to the hypothetical planet, the calculation remains the same except for the mass of the planet, which is $4M$. The gravitational force is four times greater on the hypothetical planet—or 48 N.

54. (B) To determine the equation for gravitational acceleration (g), the weight on the surface (mg) is equal to the gravitational force between an object and Earth on the surface. After canceling, the equation solves for g.

$$mg = \frac{GMm}{R^2}$$

$$g = \frac{GM}{R^2}$$

By substituting $\frac{1}{2}M$ for M and $2R$ for R—and remembering to square!—it is determined that the gravitational acceleration on the hypothetical planet is one eighth that on Earth.

55. (B) The gravitational force and gravitational acceleration—like other quantities such as intensity of light and electric force—follow the inverse square law: the quantity decreases as the inverse of the square of the factor by which distance increases. In this case, the distance doubles, and the inverse of the square of 2 is ¼. Thus, the gravitational acceleration of the new point is ¼ as great, or 0.6 m/s². (If the distance were 3 times as much, the gravitational acceleration would have been ⅑.)

56. (D) On the surface, the satellite is a distance R from the center of Earth. Its weight on the surface is $W = mg$, or 1,000 N. At the orbit insertion point, the satellite is $4R$ above the surface, five times as far from the center of Earth, so it weighs ¹⁄₂₅ as much. (The gravitational force, like many other quantities in physics, is an inverse square law, since R^2 is in the denominator of the following equation.) So the satellite weighs ¹⁄₂₅ of 1,000 N, or 40 N.

$$F_G = \frac{GMm}{R^2}$$

57. (D) The elastic potential energy of the ball and spring system is converted to kinetic energy in the ball at the instant the ball is released from the spring, which is at the equilibrium position. The spring constant, k, is solved for in the following equation, where U is elastic potential energy, K is kinetic energy, Δx is the extension of the spring from the equilibrium position when it is compressed, and Δv is the change in speed of the ball from the time the spring is released until the ball leaves the spring.

$$\Delta U_E = \Delta K$$
$$\tfrac{1}{2}k(\Delta x)^2 = \tfrac{1}{2}m(\Delta v)^2$$
$$k = \frac{m(\Delta v)^2}{\Delta x^2} = \frac{(0.1\ \text{kg})(10\ \text{m/s})^2}{(0.1\ \text{m})^2} = 1,000\ \text{N/m}$$

58. (B) When the mass is halfway between its amplitude and equilibrium positions, the displacement, x, is one half its maximum, called A (for amplitude). The potential energy at the halfway position is $\tfrac{1}{2}kx^2$, and the potential energy at its amplitude is $\tfrac{1}{2}kA^2$. When $x = \tfrac{1}{2}A$, the potential energy is one fourth the total energy at amplitude.

59. (B) The potential energy stored in a spring is $\tfrac{1}{2}kx^2$, where x is the displacement of the spring from its equilibrium position. Without a calculator, the best approach is to write out decimals as fractions and cancel: ½(200)(5/100)(5/100) = (100)(5/100)(5/100) = 25/100, or 0.25 J.

60. (A) The net external force on the system is 9 N, which is the vector sum of 12 N to the right and 3 N to the left. The total mass of the system is 6 kg, which is the total mass of all three blocks. The equation $\Sigma F = ma$ is used to solve for acceleration.

$$\vec{a} = \frac{\vec{F}}{m} = \frac{9\ \text{N}}{6\ \text{kg}} = 1.5\ \text{m/s}^2$$

Now, apply Newton's second law again—this time only on the 1 kg block.

$\Sigma \vec{F} = m\vec{a} = (1 \text{ kg})(1.5 \text{ m/s}^2) = 1.5 \text{ N}$

If the net force on the 1 kg block is 1.5 N and the friction force (to the left) on the block is 1 N, then the tension (to the right) in the string is 2.5 N.

61. (A) First, Newton's second law of motion is applied to the system of two boxes. The accelerating force is the weight of the hanging box, $mg = 100 \text{ N}$. The force acting against the motion is the friction force on the 20 kg box: $F_f = \mu N = \mu mg = (0.2)(20 \text{ kg})(10 \text{ m/s}^2) = 40 \text{ N}$. Thus, the net force on the system of two boxes is 60 N. The acceleration of the system is calculated as follows.

$$\vec{a} = \frac{\Sigma \vec{F}}{m} = \frac{60 \text{ N}}{30 \text{ kg}} = 2 \text{ m/s}^2$$

Next, Newton's second law is applied to the 10 kg mass only, using the acceleration just calculated.

$\Sigma F = mg - T = ma$

$(10 \text{ kg})(10 \text{ m/s}^2) - T = (20 \text{ kg})(2 \text{ m/s}^2)$

$100 \text{ N} - T = 40 \text{ N}$

$T = 60 \text{ N}$

62. (C) The coefficient of friction is a value less than 1, so choice (A) is incorrect. As long as the object moves across the surface, the coefficient of kinetic friction has a set value, regardless of speed, so choice (B) is incorrect. The coefficient of kinetic friction is generally considered to be less than the coefficient of static friction between an object and a surface, so choice (D) is incorrect. Rolling friction is less than sliding friction between two similar surfaces, so choice (C) is correct.

63. (B) The mass of the box is 10 kg if the weight of the box on Earth is 100 N, since $W = mg$. Newton's second law of motion is applied.

$\Sigma F = ma$

$F_{pulling} - F_{friction} = ma$

$30 \text{ N} - F_{friction} = (10 \text{ kg})(2 \text{ m/s}^2)$

$F_{friction} = 10 \text{ N}$

If the box is pulled at constant speed, the net force would be zero, and the friction force would be equal to the pulling force.

64. (A) As the angle of the ramp is increased, the normal force of the ramp on the box decreases. (When the ramp becomes vertical, the gravitational force on the box is also vertical, so the box does not exert any normal force on the ramp—and by Newton's third law, the ramp does not exert any normal force on the box.) The friction force depends on the coefficient of friction and the normal force. If the normal force decreases as the ramp is tilted, then the friction between the two surfaces also decreases.

65. (C) Let's talk this one through, using a "system approach." By Newton's second law, the net force on the system of boxes must be enough to accelerate the boxes. The system of boxes has a mass of 6 kg, so the net force must be equal to mass times acceleration (ma), or 3 N. The friction force on the boxes is equal to the coefficient of friction times the normal force of the surface on the boxes. Since the surface is level, the normal force is equal to the weight of the boxes ($F_N = mg = 60$ N). The friction force is equal to μF_N, or 6 N. Since the net force must be 3 N (see above), the pulling force must be 9 N.

$$F_{pulling} - F_{friction} = ma$$
$$9 \text{ N} - 6 \text{ N} = (6 \text{ kg})(0.5 \text{ m/s}^2)$$

66. (A) As the parachutist falls due to the force of gravity exerted on her, velocity increases. However, as the velocity increases, the friction force of air (air drag) increases. Once the friction force increases to the point that the friction force upward on the parachutist is equal to the gravitational force downward, the parachutist is in equilibrium—since there is no longer a net force—and there is no longer an acceleration. The parachutist then falls at a constant velocity, called terminal velocity. Choice (A) is true. In choice (B), if the gravitational force is greater than the friction force of air, then the parachutist is not only falling downward but still accelerating downward, so she is not falling at terminal velocity. Choice (C) cannot be true at terminal velocity, because if the friction force, which is upward, is greater than the gravitational force, the parachutist would be accelerating upward. Choice (D) cannot be true, because as long as the parachutist is moving through air (that is, falling), there is a friction force of air on her.

67. (C) To start the box moving, the pulling force must be just large enough to overcome the friction force, which is equal to 40 N. The normal force, assuming a level surface, is equal to the weight of the box, which is mg. At this point, the equation $F_F = \mu F_N$ is used to solve for the coefficient of friction.

$$\mu = \frac{F_F}{F_N} = \frac{40 \text{ N}}{mg} = \frac{40 \text{ N}}{100 \text{ N}} = 0.40$$

68. (C) Use the formula $F_F = \mu F_N$ to determine the values for the friction force and the normal force. Since the box is sliding at constant speed, this is an equilibrium situation and therefore the sum of forces in each direction is zero. For frame of reference, set the x axis parallel to the incline and the y axis perpendicular to the incline. The forces parallel to the incline must add to zero, so the friction force, F_F, is equal to the force component 20 sin 40°. The forces perpendicular to the surface must also be equal to each other, so the normal force, F_N, is equal to 20 cos 40°.

$$\mu = \frac{F_F}{F_N} = \frac{20 \sin 40°}{20 \cos 40°}$$

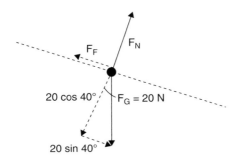

20 cos 40° $F_G = 20$ N

20 sin 40°

69. (C) Since the applied force is three times farther from the fulcrum than the box is from the fulcrum, the force needs to be only one third the weight of the box in order to balance it or move it at constant speed (both equilibrium conditions). However, the input work and output work must be the same, according to conservation of energy principles.

$$W_{input} = W_{output}$$
$$F_{input}d_{input} = F_{output}d_{output}$$

If the input force, F, is one third the output force (or weight of the box), then the input distance must be three times the output distance. Each end of the board changes position in the same amount of time, so the input force must move three times as far in the same amount of time—and is moving three times as fast.

70. (B) The bottom pulley is a single movable pulley, which has a mechanical advantage of 2. (The tension throughout the rope must be the same, and there are two parts of rope supporting the weight of the object.) Therefore, each rope part at the bottom pulley is supporting one half the weight of the object, and the tension in each part of the rope is $\frac{1}{2}W$. That is, the tension in the rope pulling downward—and the force F—is $\frac{1}{2}W$. The upper pulley has a mechanical advantage of 1. It simply changes the direction of the force and does not multiply the force.

The total mechanical advantage is the product of the mechanical advantage of each pulley, which is 1×2, or 2. This pulley system multiplies the input force by 2 and is able to lift twice as much as the input force; therefore, again, $W = 2F$.

Energy must be conserved, and work input must equal work output, assuming no frictional losses in the pulleys. Since work equals force times distance and the input force is one half the output force (weight lifted), the input force must move twice as far as the object is lifted.

$$W_{input} = W_{output}$$
$$F_{input}d_{input} = F_{output}d_{output}$$

71. (B) The weight of the object is mg. The mechanical advantage of the movable pulley, which is attached to the object, is 2. (There are two tension forces upward on the pulley, and one gravitational force downward.) Lifting the object at constant speed is an equilibrium situation, that is, the net force is zero, since there is no acceleration. Therefore, each of the rope parts at the movable pulley is pulling upward with one half the weight of the object. The single fixed pulley attached to the ceiling has a mechanical advantage of 1, since it only changes the direction of the force. The total mechanical advantage of the pulley system is the product of the mechanical advantages of the individual pulleys, which is 1×2, or 2. This means that the pulley system multiplies the input effort by 2, enabling the operator of the machine to use one half the force that is being moved.

Remember that the tension throughout the rope must be the same, assuming that the weight of the rope is ignored. If the person pulls downward with $\frac{1}{2}mg$, the tension in each part of the rope at the movable pulley is also $\frac{1}{2}mg$, but there are two of them pulling upward. Therefore, the $\frac{1}{2}mg$ effort on the right can lift the mg on the left.

72. (C) The single fixed pulley attached to the tree limb has a mechanical advantage of 1; it only changes the direction of the force. The weight of the children is 400 N ($W = mg$), so the father must pull downward with a force of 400 N to lift them at constant speed. Recognize that constant speed is an equilibrium situation where the net force is zero (that is, there is no acceleration), so the force pulling upward on the children is equal in magnitude to the gravitational force downward.

Chapter 3: Gravitation and Circular Motion

73. (A) The gravitational acceleration g on the surface of any planet is directly proportional to the mass of the planet and inversely proportional to the radius of the planet squared (since the radius of the planet is the distance between the planet and any object on its surface). The mass of the object on the surface does not affect the value of g. The equation describing this relationship can be derived by setting the weight of any object on the surface, mg, equal to the gravitational force between the planet (of mass M) and the object (of mass m), where R is the radius of the planet.

$$mg = \frac{GMm}{R^2}$$

$$g = \frac{GM}{R^2}$$

74. (C) The new location of the object is twice as far from the center of Earth as it had been on the surface. Since the gravitational force and gravitational field follow inverse square laws, the object would weigh one fourth as much as it does on the surface; that is, the distance, which is twice as great, is squared to get 4, and the new quantity is the inverse of that, or one fourth as much. Many quantities in physics, such as light intensity, sound intensity, electric force, and electric field, follow inverse square laws with distance.

75. (A) Though the object would, indeed, weigh one sixth as much on the surface of the moon as it does on Earth, the mass of the object would not change.

76. (B) Due to its motion in a circle on the rotating Earth, an object on the surface has a centripetal force equal to the quantity mv^2/R, which is provided by the gravitational force toward the center of Earth—the gravitational force of Earth on the object. However, since Earth rotates, an object on the surface is constantly accelerating centripetally and is therefore not in an inertial frame of reference. In this accelerating frame of reference, the object is trying to move outward, seeming to experience a centrifugal force that decreases the net force toward the center of Earth. (Note that this outward force exists only in a noninertial frame of reference.) Thus, the effective value of g decreases slightly. In choice (A), the sun and moon would each, at times, exert gravitational force on the object away from the center of Earth, decreasing the net force on the object; however, since Earth, the sun, and the moon change positions relative to each other as Earth and moon orbit, this effect would not be consistently less.

77. (C) The value for the gravitational field, g, for the smaller planet is calculated using the following equation.

$$g_{small} = \frac{GM}{R^2}$$

The larger planet has a radius three times the radius of the smaller planet, so its volume is 27 times the volume of the smaller planet. (The volume of a sphere is $4/3\pi R^3$.) Since the planets have the same density, the ratio of mass/volume must be the same for both planets; thus, the larger planet must also have 27 times the mass of the smaller planet. These values are substituted to calculate the value of g for the larger planet.

$$g_{large} = \frac{G(27M)}{(3R)^2} = \frac{3GM}{R^2}$$

Since the larger planet has three times the value of g, the object will weigh three times as much on the surface of the larger planet, or 90 N.

78. (D) The equation for gravitational force is used, where M is the mass of Earth, m is the mass of the object, and R is the radius of Earth. The mass of the sun is 300,000M, and the radius of the sun is 100R.

$$F_{earth} = \frac{GMm}{R^2}$$

$$F_{sun} = \frac{G(300,000M)m}{(100R)^2} = \frac{30GMm}{R^2}$$

79. (A) Density is equal to mass divided by volume. Since object A and object B have the same radius, they have the same volume. Therefore, object A, with twice the density, must have twice the mass of object B. In the formula for calculating the gravitational force between objects A and C or between objects B and C, the force between objects B and C will be twice as large.

80. (D) First, the net gravitational force on object A, due to the other two objects, will be the sum of the force of B on A and the force of C on A, and the force will be to the right. Second, the magnitude of the net gravitational force on object C is the same, since both objects A and B are attracting object C to the left—and the same sets of numbers in the gravitational force equation would be used for the calculation. Third, the net gravitational force on object B is less than the others, since object A is attracting object B to the left and object C is attracting object B to the right. To determine the net force on object B, the forces of the other two objects on object B are subtracted, since the net force is the sum of vectors in the opposite direction.

81. (A) First, the 4 kg object located at $x = 6$ has four times the mass of the object at $x = 0$. The distance between objects in the formula shown is squared, so doubling the distance in the denominator and squaring it would cancel the quadrupled mass in the numerator. This means that the magnitude of the force on the 3 kg object due to the 4 kg object would be equal to the magnitude of the force on the 3 kg object due to the 1 kg object if the 4 kg object were twice as far away from the 3 kg object. Positioning the 3 kg object at $x = 2$ would accomplish this. By substituting in the formula below, it is determined that the two quantities would be equal.

$$F_G = \frac{GMm}{R^2}$$

$$F_{4 \text{ kg on B}} = \frac{G(4 \text{ kg})(3 \text{ kg})}{(4 \text{ units})^2}$$

$$F_{1 \text{ kg on B}} = \frac{G(1 \text{ kg})(3 \text{ kg})}{(2 \text{ units})^2}$$

82. (D) When the satellite is in orbit, the distance between Earth and the satellite (used in the gravitational formula to calculate force) is 4 Earth radii. The altitude above the surface must be added to the radius of Earth to determine the total distance between them. When the satellite is on the surface of Earth, this orbital radius is four times the distance. Since the gravitational force follows an inverse square relationship, the force on the satellite in orbit is $(\frac{1}{4})^2$, or one sixteenth the force that Earth exerts on the satellite when it is on the surface.

83. (A) According to Newton's third law of motion, the force that one object exerts on a second object is equal in magnitude to the force that the second object exerts on the first object.

84. (B) Once the satellite is moving in a stable circular orbit, only Earth's gravitational force is required to provide the centripetal force. Choice (A) is incorrect, because without any force exerted on the satellite, it would take a linear path due to its own inertia (which is not a force). Choice (C) is incorrect, because the satellite would move tangentially in its orbit due to its own inertia. Choice (D) is incorrect, because the gravitational force of Earth on the satellite provides the centripetal force to keep the satellite moving in a circle; there is no additional centripetal force.

85. (D) The gravitational force of Earth on the satellite provides the centripetal force to keep the satellite in orbit. This fact is used to derive an equation for the velocity of the satellite in orbit as a function of the distance R between the center of the satellite and the center of Earth.

$$\frac{GM_{Earth}m_{satellite}}{R_{orbit}^2} = \frac{m_{satellite}v^2}{R_{orbit}}$$

$$v = \sqrt{\frac{GM}{R}}$$

The original value for orbital radius R is a total of four Earth radii—three Earth radii above the surface plus one Earth radius to the center. If the new speed of the satellite is one half as much, the value of R inside the radical must be four times greater, so that taking the square root makes v equal to one half as much. The new orbital radius, then, must be four times that of the original—or 16 Earth radii from the center of Earth—definitely more than four Earth radii above the surface.

86. (C) For the speed of the object to remain constant, the centripetal force must be constant, since centripetal force is equal to mv^2/R, assuming that the mass and radius will be constant in the circular path. At the top of the circle, the centripetal force is provided by the tension in the string and the weight of the object—both toward the center of the circle. At the bottom of the circle, the tension is toward the center and the weight of the object is away from the center, so the tension must be greater. At the bottom, the tension is providing the centripetal force *and* holding the object from falling downward due to its own weight. It is possible for the tension to be zero, as in choice (D), since the weight of the object provides the centripetal force at the top of the motion, but it does not have to be zero.

87. (C) The centripetal force is provided by a force toward the center of the turn. Both the gravitational forces and the normal forces are perpendicular to the surface, so they are both perpendicular to the radius of the turn and do not provide the centripetal force. Inertia is not a force. As the automobile turns the corner, its attempted motion is along a tangent outward, so the friction force opposes that motion—inward toward the center, providing the centripetal force to keep the automobile in the turn.

88. (D) When the string is cut, the ball will take a parabolic path at the speed of 1 m/s as it falls to the floor, gaining vertical speed due to the gravitational force exerted on it. The ball will then hit the floor at a speed greater than 1 m/s.

89. (D) The minimum speed at the top of the vertical circle for ball A is the speed at which the weight (mg) of the ball alone provides the centripetal force. For the speed to be minimum, the tension in the string must be zero, and the speed is determined as follows.

$$mg = \frac{mv^2}{R}$$

$$v = \sqrt{gR}$$

Since student B has a string that is $2R$, the speed is $\sqrt{2}$ times that of ball A, even without any tension in the string. Adding tension in the string will only increase the speed, so none of the conditions in choices (A) through (C) will allow student B to match the speed of ball A.

90. (B) Assuming that the nickel is moving at constant speed in the circle, its speed is equal to the distance around the circle ($2\pi R$) divided by the time for each circle (1 s).

$$v = \frac{2\pi R}{t} = \frac{2\pi (0.10 \text{ m})}{1 \text{ s}} = 0.2\pi \text{ m/s}$$

91. (A) The gravitational force between Earth and the satellite is set equal to the expression for centripetal force. (The distance used in both formulas must be the total distance from center to center, which is $R + h$.)

$$\frac{GMm}{(R + h)^2} = \frac{mv^2}{R + h}$$

$$\frac{GM}{R + h} = v^2$$

92. (D) Creating a banked curve higher on the outside allows a component of the normal force of the road on a vehicle to be directed toward the center of the curve, increasing the force centripetally. Choice (A) is not the most effective measure, because smaller vehicles will still not be able to negotiate the curve; appropriate speed does not depend on the mass of the vehicle (since mass cancels in the calculations). Choice (B) is not correct, because banking so that the road is higher on the inside actually increases the problem. If the road is lower on the outside of the curve, a component of the normal force is directed outward. Choice (C) is not correct, because decreasing the radius increases the centripetal force necessary to keep a vehicle on the road ($F = mv^2/R$).

93. (B) At the equator, the radius of the circle on which the location is rotating is the radius of Earth. At 60° of latitude, the distance to the center of Earth is approximately the same, but the circle on which the location is moving is one half the distance to the axis of rotation, as shown.

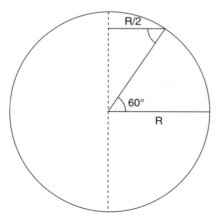

The time for one complete rotation is the same everywhere, but reducing the radius of the circle to one half also decreases the speed to one half.

94. (C) To examine the factors that affect the washer as it moves in a circle, it is important to remember that it is the friction force of the turntable surface on the washer that provides the centripetal force.

$$F_F = F_C$$

$$\mu mg = \frac{mv^2}{R}$$

$$v = \sqrt{\mu gR}$$

As can be seen from the equation, mass is not a factor, so stacking washers or reducing the mass of the washer, as in choices (A) and (B), would have no effect. In choice (C), scratching the bottom of the washer to make it rougher would increase the coefficient of friction between the turntable and washer surfaces.

95. (B) As the pendulum oscillates, the tension force on the object is directed toward the center of the arc and the gravitational force is directed downward toward the floor. Since the pendulum has its maximum speed at the bottom of its swing (when gravitational potential energy has been converted to kinetic energy), the tension is maximum. The tension at the bottom of the pendulum's swing (see the illustration at left) is equal to the weight of the object on the string plus the centripetal force necessary to keep the object moving in a circle at that velocity. The tension cannot be constant, as in choice (A), because the speed is changing and the direction of the gravitational force on the object is also changing. In the illustration at right, the tension is equal to the component of the gravitational force opposite (which is less than mg) plus the centripetal force, which is also less, because the speed is less.

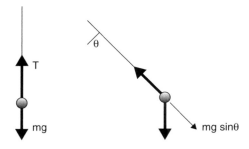

At the bottom of the swing, the following formula applies.

$$T - mg = \frac{mv^2}{R}$$

When the pendulum is at an angle, v is less and $mg \sin \theta$ is less than mg, and the following formula applies.

$$T - mg \sin \theta = \frac{mv^2}{R}$$

96. (C) Choice (A) is true, because the centripetal force on the satellite is, by definition, toward the center of the orbit in order to keep the satellite moving in a circle. Choice (B) is true by Newton's third law of motion: for every action there is an equal and opposite action on another object. Choice (D) is true, because there is a constant centripetal acceleration, that is, a change in direction of the velocity vector as the satellite moves in a circle. Choice (C) is not true, for the same reason that choice (B) is true.

97. (A) The forces on the small object inside the cone are shown: mg downward, a normal force perpendicular to the inside surface, and friction upward along the inside surface opposing the attempted slide of the object downward. The only force directed toward the center of the circle in which the object is moving would be a component of the normal force, as described in choice (A).

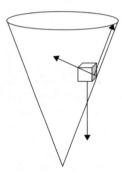

98. (C) If the object moves at constant speed in the circle and the angle remains constant, there is an equilibrium (that is, no acceleration) in the vertical direction and, therefore, the net force on the object in the vertical direction must be zero. There are only two forces on the object in the vertical direction: the gravitational force on the object downward (mg, or $0.25 \text{ kg} \times g$) and the component of the tension in the string that is upward, $T \cos 60°$.

99. (C) By Newton's universal law of gravitation, any two objects in the universe exert forces of equal magnitude on each other. Thus, the moon exerts the same force on Earth as Earth exerts on the moon, with the forces along a line between their centers and in opposite directions.

100. (B) For the value of gravitational acceleration, g, to be less, the shuttle must be farther from Earth. The gravitational force is equal to the weight of the shuttle, mg.

$$\frac{GM_{\text{Earth}}m_{\text{satellite}}}{R_{\text{orbit}}^2} = mg$$

$$g = \frac{GM_{\text{Earth}}}{R_{\text{orbit}}^2}$$

Next to be determined is the relationship between the speed of the shuttle in its orbit and the distance of the shuttle from Earth. The gravitational force provides the centripetal force for the shuttle's circular orbit.

$$\frac{GM_{\text{Earth}}m_{\text{satellite}}}{R_{\text{orbit}}^2} = \frac{m_{\text{satellite}}v^2}{R_{\text{orbit}}}$$

$$v = \sqrt{\frac{GM}{R}}$$

For the orbital radius to be greater (providing a lower value of g), orbital speed must be less.

101. (B) In a circular orbit, speed is simply distance divided by time. The distance is the circumference of a circle, 2π times the radius, and the time for each orbit is the period, T. It is crucial to remember that the radius of the orbit is the center-to-center distance, which is the radius of Earth plus the distance of the space debris from Earth (assuming that the radius of the space debris itself is negligible).

$$v = \frac{\text{distance}}{\text{time}} = \frac{2\pi(R + r)}{T}$$

102. (C) A force toward the center of the arc of the curve would provide the centripetal force necessary for the car to move in a circle. The gravitational force, or weight of the car, is toward the center of Earth, so choice (A) is incorrect. Since there is no friction force due to the ice, choice (B) is incorrect. Inertia is not a force; as a matter of fact, inertia describes the tendency of the car to move in a straight line off the curve if there is no centripetal force. A free-body diagram of the car on the banked surface shows that the normal force is perpendicular to the surface with one vertical component that is equal to the weight of the car and one horizontal component inward toward the center of the circle (the centripetal force).

103. (B) Essentially, this is an application of Newton's second law of motion, with the net force equal to the sum of the tension force toward the center of the circle (that is, upward) and the weight of the stone away from the circle (that is, downward). The acceleration is the centripetal acceleration.

$$\Sigma F = ma$$

$$T - mg = \frac{mv^2}{R}$$

$$120 - mg = \frac{mv^2}{1.2}$$

104. (D) It is not necessary to know the mass of the object in the calculation of its centripetal acceleration.

$$a_{\text{center}} = \frac{v^2}{R} = \frac{(20 \text{ m/s})^2}{100 \text{ m}} = 4 \text{ m/s}^2$$

105. (B) It is not necessary to know the mass of the car in the calculation of its centripetal acceleration (v^2/R). When radius and speed are both doubled, the speed is squared in the numerator, so the new acceleration is 4/2, or 2, times greater.

106. (A) The net force at the bottom of the stone's path is the difference between the tension, T, upward and the weight of the rock, mg, downward. This net force can be determined using Newton's second law; the acceleration in this case is the centripetal acceleration.

$$\Sigma F = T - mg = ma$$

$$T - mg = \frac{mv^2}{R}$$

$$T = (2 \text{ kg})(10 \text{ m/s}^2) + \frac{(2 \text{ kg})(4 \text{ m/s})^2}{0.5} = 20 + 64 = 84 \text{ N}$$

107. (B) The centripetal force equation is used: $F = mv^2/R$. If the radius is doubled, the force must be half as much.

108. (B) An object traveling in a circle at constant speed is constantly changing direction, so its velocity (which is a vector) is not constant. If the object is traveling at constant speed, it has no tangential acceleration—only an inward radial (that is, centripetal) acceleration.

109. (B) If the two satellites are in orbits at different distances from Earth, they must be moving at different speeds. Since the force providing the centripetal force must be the gravitational force, the two expressions are set equal to each other to determine the relationship between velocity and orbital radius.

$$\frac{GM_{\text{Earth}}m_{\text{satellite}}}{R_{\text{orbit}}^2} = \frac{m_{\text{satellite}}v^2}{R_{\text{orbit}}}$$

$$v = \sqrt{\frac{GM}{R}}$$

The speed in orbit, v, is inversely proportional to the orbital radius, so the satellite orbiting nearer to Earth must be moving faster. Applying the formula for centripetal acceleration, $a = v^2/R$, the centripetal acceleration must get larger as orbital radius is reduced. The masses of the satellites cancel and are not factors in the calculations.

Chapter 4: Linear Momentum

110. (D) Momentum, p, is equal to mv, and kinetic energy, K, is equal to $\frac{1}{2}mv^2$. Assuming that the mass of the object remains constant, doubling the momentum causes the velocity to double. Since the velocity term in K is squared, doubling the velocity would make the kinetic energy four times greater than before. This can be easily understood by deriving an expression for kinetic energy in terms of momentum. Doubling momentum quadruples kinetic energy.

$$p = mv$$

$$v = \frac{p}{m}$$

$$K = \frac{1}{2}mv^2 = \frac{1}{2}m\left(\frac{p}{m}\right)^2 = \frac{p^2}{2m}$$

111. (D) Change in momentum, Δp, is equal to $m\Delta v$, as long as mass remains constant. When this formula is applied in choice (D), the result is $m\Delta v/m$, or Δv. Choice (A) would be equal to $m\Delta v/t$, which is the rate of change in momentum or force. Choice (B) is force times time, which is the change in momentum, or impulse. Choice (C) is equal to force over time and therefore not equal to change in velocity.

112. (C) Assuming that all motion is in one dimension on the air track, one momentum equation can show conservation of momentum during the collision of the carts. First, the momenta, $p = mv$, for the two carts are added. Then, the momentum to the right is set as positive and the momentum to the left as negative. Before the collision, the net momentum is $(2)(1) + (1)(-3)$, or a net of -1. Therefore, the momentum after the collision must also be -1. The 2 kg cart has a momentum of -4 kg·m/s, so the 1 kg cart must have a momentum of $+3$ for the momenta to add to -1. Thus, the 1 kg cart must be moving at 3 m/s to the right.

$$\Sigma p_o = \Sigma p_f$$
$$m_1 v_{1o} + m_2 v_{2o} = m_1 v_{1f} + m_2 v_{2f}$$
$$(2 \text{ kg})(1 \text{ m/s}) + (1 \text{ kg})(-3 \text{ m/s}) = (2 \text{ kg})(-2 \text{ m/s}) + (1 \text{ kg})(v)$$
$$v = 3 \text{ m/s}$$

113. (D) In a totally inelastic collision, the colliding objects stick together to form one object. Even though kinetic energy is not conserved in an inelastic collision, it can be assumed that momentum is conserved. Considering the velocity to the right positive and the velocity to the left negative, the net momentum before the collision is $2mv + -4mv$, or $-2mv$. Therefore, the net momentum after the collision must be $-2mv$. The combined objects after the collision have a mass of $2m$, so the velocity of the objects afterward must be $-v$, which is to the left.

$$\Sigma p_o = \Sigma p_f$$
$$m_1 v_{1o} + m_2 v_{2o} = (m_1 + m_2)v_f$$
$$m(2v) + m(-4v) = 2mv_f$$
$$v_f = -v$$

114. (D) Since the skaters are on ice, there is no friction on the skaters, and in the absence of an external force on the two skaters, linear momentum will be conserved. The momentum before they push off each other is zero; therefore, the total momentum after they start moving must be zero. They must move in opposite directions so that the sum of their momenta—one negative and one positive—is still zero.

$$p_o = p_f$$
$$0 = m_1 v_1 + m_2 v_2$$
$$0 = (40 \text{ kg})v_1 + (50 \text{ kg})v_2$$
$$\frac{v_1}{v_2} = -\frac{5}{4}$$

115. (C) By Newton's second law of motion, force is equal to the rate of change in momentum: $F = \Delta p/\Delta t = m\Delta v/\Delta t$. If the mass of the cart is the same both times and the contact time is the same both times, the force would be proportional to the change in velocity. For an elastic collision, the final velocity is the negative of the initial velocity (since it is in the opposite direction): $-2v$. If the initial velocity is doubled, the force exerted on the wall is doubled.

116. (C) This is a totally inelastic collision, where momentum is conserved but kinetic energy is not conserved. It is unnecessary to know the mass of each cart, as their masses will cancel in the solution. The conservation of linear momentum is determined.

$$p_o = p_f$$
$$m_1 v_1 + 0 = (m_1 + m_2)v_2$$
$$m(2 \text{ m/s}) + 0 = (2m)v_2$$
$$v_2 = 1 \text{ m/s}$$

117. (B) Chart A indicates that the initial velocity of cart A is about $+1.2$ m/s and its final velocity is about -2.2 m/s. The collision contact starts at $t = 0.3$ s and ends at $t = 0.7$ s, so the time of contact is 0.4 s. The force is calculated as the rate of change in momentum.

$$F = \frac{\Delta p}{\Delta t} = \frac{m(v_{\text{final}} - v_{\text{initial}})}{t} = \frac{(1 \text{ kg})(-2.2 \text{ m/s} - 1.2 \text{ m/s})}{0.4 \text{ s}} = \frac{-3.4}{0.4} = -8.5 \text{ N}$$

Chart B indicates that the initial velocity of cart B is about $+2.2$ m/s and its final velocity is about -1.2 m/s, so the change in velocity is the same. The two carts have exchanged velocities—and exerted equal and opposite forces on each other. (Note: Since the motion sensors face each other, a positive velocity for sensor A is in the same direction as a negative velocity for sensor B; that is, velocity away from the sensor is recorded as positive.)

118. (C) Change in momentum is impulse, but the rate at which momentum changes is force. Essentially, this is a statement of Newton's second law of motion.

$$F = \frac{\Delta p}{\Delta t}$$

119. (B) The area under the graph line is the change in momentum, $m\Delta v$, which is called impulse. The impulse is equal to force times time, $F\Delta t$ ($F\Delta t = \Delta p$). The area above the graph line is a triangle, with area $= \frac{1}{2}bh$. To find the area, the time of contact is multiplied by $\frac{1}{2}$ times the maximum force, which is average force. It is important to note that the racket exerts the same force on the ball that the ball exerts on the racket, and the ball and racket also exert equal and opposite impulses on each other.

$$F = \frac{\Delta p}{\Delta t}$$
$$F\Delta t = \Delta p$$

120. (A) Newton's second law of motion is applied. The change in momentum is the same in both situations, the car's mass remains the same, and the initial and final velocities are the same. Therefore, reducing the time by half means that the force applied to stop the car must be doubled.

$$F = \frac{\Delta p}{\Delta t}$$

$$F\Delta t = \Delta p$$

121. (A) Newton's second law of motion can be stated in terms of change in momentum.

$$\Sigma F = \frac{\Delta p}{\Delta t}$$

The automobile's momentum change will be the same regardless of time, that is, from momentum mv to momentum equal to zero when it stops. The key to less force on the occupants during the stop is increasing the time—which decreases force. An air bag increases the stopping time of the person who moves into the bag after it is deployed. Choice (B) is not correct, because the person does not move as far when an air bag is in place (although the second part, decreasing acceleration, would be helpful). Choice (C) is not correct, because the softness of the air bag doesn't explain the physics in terms of increased time and reduced force. Choice (D) implies that large forces in opposite directions on a person would yield a net force of zero—but that is not logical.

122. (C) The area under the graph is the change in momentum of the object ($Ft = m\Delta v$). Assuming that the forward motion of the object toward the wall is the positive direction and, therefore, the change in momentum and change in velocity are in the negative direction, dividing by the mass of the object will yield the change in velocity.

$$F = \frac{m\Delta v}{\Delta t}$$

$$\Delta v = \frac{F\Delta t}{m} = \frac{\text{Area}}{m} = \frac{\frac{1}{2}(5\ \text{N})(1.0 \times 10^{-3}\ \text{s})}{0.25\ \text{kg}} = 0.01\ \text{m/s}$$

123. (C) Assuming that the time of contact between the ball and the target is about the same for both throws, and assuming a nearly elastic collision so that the ball rebounds at about the same speed as it hit, doubling the speed of the throw will double the force on the target.

$$F = \frac{m\Delta v}{\Delta t} = \frac{m(v_f - v_o)}{\Delta t} = \frac{m(-v_o - v_o)}{\Delta t} = -\frac{2mv_o}{\Delta t}$$

$$F' = \frac{m\Delta v}{\Delta t} = \frac{m(2v_f - 2v_o)}{\Delta t} = \frac{m(-2v_o - 2v_o)}{\Delta t} = -\frac{4mv_o}{\Delta t} = -4F$$

Since the force of the target on the ball is negative, the force of the ball on the target is positive.

124. (A) If there are no external forces, then linear momentum is conserved. However, if the collision were totally inelastic, then the objects would stick together on impact and part of the kinetic energy would convert to thermal energy of the objects. Kinetic energy is not conserved in inelastic collisions.

125. (A) Linear momentum depends on both mass and velocity: $p = mv$. If either of these quantities changes, momentum changes. Thus, velocity could remain constant while the mass of the system changes, producing a change in momentum.

126. (A) In an elastic collision, both momentum and kinetic energy are conserved. In an inelastic collision, however, only momentum is conserved—kinetic energy is not conserved. In a totally inelastic collision, kinetic energy is not conserved and the colliding objects stick together during the collision.

127. (C) In an elastic collision between two particles of equal mass, there are several possibilities: (1) If one particle is stationary and the other particle hits it head-on, the second particle will transfer its momentum to the first particle, so the second particle stops in the position of the first particle. (2) If both particles are moving when they collide head-on, they will exchange speeds. (3) If one particle is initially stationary and a second particle hits it off-center (as in the example given), the two particles will move off at right angles to each other. Their speeds are not necessarily equal—they would be equal only if each particle moves off at an angle of 45° to its original direction of motion. The proof of this last case is not difficult, because when the conservation of kinetic energy equation is written, the masses cancel to leave a Pythagorean relationship between the velocities: $v^2 = v_1^2 + v_2^2$.

128. (A) Kinetic energy is lost during a collision in the sense that the energy is converted to another form of energy, such as thermal energy of the molecules of the colliding object, or to sound or light. For example, when two objects collide, the sound of the collision may be heard. That sound energy, which is actually thermal energy of molecules, comes from kinetic energy of the moving objects prior to the collision, so the objects have less kinetic energy after the collision. This is the definition of an inelastic collision. Momentum is conserved, but kinetic energy is not conserved.

129. (B) When two moving objects collide head-on and elastically, the motion will all be along a line (that is, in one dimension) and both momentum and kinetic energy will be conserved during the collision. Because the objects are of equal mass, they will cancel during the derivation and only their velocities need to be considered. Choice (A) is not correct, because kinetic energy is conserved during elastic collisions, and in this case there would be no kinetic energy after the collision. Choice (C) is impossible in the situation where one object is moving faster than the other prior to collision; it could not collide and retain its velocity, since that would imply that it is moving in the same direction at the same speed after hitting another object. Choice (D) is not correct, because if the objects collide head-on, the motion would be entirely in one dimension.

130. (A) If the collision of the photon causes the electron to move with kinetic energy K, then in order to conserve momentum and mass energy, the photon must have less energy. A photon with less energy has a lower frequency and longer wavelength ($E = hf = hc/\lambda$). This is called the Compton effect; the emitted photon comes off at an angle called the Compton angle, and it can be shown that the components of momentum for the electron and emitted photon will add to zero so that momentum is also conserved.

131. (D) First, the force exerted by the rubber ball will be greater than the force exerted by the dart. Force equals the rate of change in momentum. For the dart, the change in momentum is from mv to zero. For the elastic ball, the change in momentum is from mv to $-mv$, so the change in momentum is $-2mv$ — twice the change in momentum as the dart and with twice the force. Next, hitting the block of wood at the top exerts more torque on the block (force times distance from the pivot, which is at the bottom of the block). Hitting the block with the elastic ball near the top of the block is most likely to knock it over.

132. (C) Coefficient of restitution (e) describes the ratio of velocity after two objects collide to the ratio of velocity before they collide. The floor doesn't move a measurable amount due to the collision, so the ratio of v_{after} to v_{before} for the ball is used determine the coefficient. Those velocities are not provided, but the heights given help determine the velocities, using conservation of mechanical energy. When the ball is dropped, its gravitational potential energy is converted to the kinetic energy that the ball has when it hits the floor. Also, the kinetic energy the ball has after it hits the floor is converted to gravitational potential energy when the ball rises again to its maximum height. Either conversion can be used to derive an expression for velocity.

$$e = \frac{-v_{after}}{v_{before}} = \frac{-v_2}{v_1} = \frac{-\sqrt{2gh_2}}{\sqrt{2gh_1}} = \sqrt{\frac{h_2}{h_1}}$$

Since the initial and final velocities are in opposite directions, the velocities have opposite signs. The negative sign in the formula for e assures that the value of e is positive.

133. (A) Newton's second law is used to solve for v.

$$F = \frac{m\Delta v}{\Delta t} = \frac{m(v - v_o)}{t}$$

$$F = mv - mv_o$$

$$v = \frac{Ft + mv_o}{m} = \frac{Ft}{m} + v_o$$

134. (D) The center of mass of the rocket will continue to follow the path described by the first launch, which is 30 m forward from the launch site. When the rocket splits into two pieces, there is no net external force in the horizontal direction, so momentum is conserved in the direction of motion. Therefore, if the larger piece has momentum mv and lands 3 m short of the predicted (center of mass) landing site, then the smaller piece, with momentum $\frac{1}{2}mv$, would land twice as far on the other side of the predicted (center of mass) landing site, so the smaller piece lands 6 m farther, or 36 m forward from the launch site.

135. (C) Linear momentum must be conserved in each dimension. Before the collision, the only momentum is in the positive x direction, with no momentum in the y direction. After the collision, ball 2 has a momentum component in the negative y direction, so ball 1 must have a momentum component in the positive y direction, and therefore the sum is still zero. Only choice (C) has a momentum component in the positive y direction.

136. (C) Conservation of mechanical energy is used, with the gravitational potential energy (U) before the ball is dropped equal to the kinetic energy (K) just before the ball hits the floor, to determine the velocity (v_o) before the ball hits the floor the first time.

$$\Delta U = \Delta K$$

$$mgH = \tfrac{1}{2}mv_o^2$$

$$v_o = \sqrt{2gh}$$

Next, the coefficient of restitution is used to compare the velocities before and after the ball hits the floor, with velocity afterward equal to $-v_o$.

$$e = 0.5 = -\frac{v_f}{v_o} = \frac{v}{\sqrt{2gH}}$$

$$v = \tfrac{1}{2}\sqrt{2gH}$$

Then, the velocity when H is quadrupled is determined.

$$v_{new} = \tfrac{1}{2}\sqrt{2g(4H)} = \sqrt{2gH}$$

This value is twice the original velocity after the collision.

137. (C) In elastic collisions of two objects of equal mass, the objects exchange velocities; therefore, choice (C) is correct. The following proof shows that (1) linear momentum is conserved and (2) that kinetic energy is conserved.

(1) $p_o = p_f$

$$mv_{oA} + mv_{oB} = mv_{fA} + mv_{fB}$$

The equal masses are canceled, and substitutions are made.

$$v_{oA} + v_{oB} = v_{fA} + v_{fB}$$

$$(6 \text{ m/s}) + (-4 \text{ m/s}) = v_{fA} + v_{fB}$$

$$v_{fA} = 2 \text{ m/s} - v_{fB}$$

(2) $K_o = K_f$

$$\tfrac{1}{2}mv_{oA}^2 + \tfrac{1}{2}mv_{oB}^2 = \tfrac{1}{2}mv_{fA}^2 + \tfrac{1}{2}mv_{fB}^2$$

The equal masses are canceled, and substitutions are made.

$$\tfrac{1}{2}v_{oA}^2 + \tfrac{1}{2}v_{oB}^2 = \tfrac{1}{2}v_{fA}^2 + \tfrac{1}{2}v_{fB}^2$$

$$(6 \text{ m/s})^2 + (-4 \text{ m/s})^2 = v_{fA}^2 + v_{fB}^2$$

$$52 - (-2 - v_{fB})^2 = v_{fB}^2$$

$$52 - 4 + 4v_{fB} - v_{fB}^2 = v_{fB}^2$$

$$2v_{fB}^2 - 4v_{fB} - 48 = 0$$

$v_{FB}^2 - 2v_{FB} - 24 = 0$

$(v_{FB} - 6)(v_{FB} + 4) = 0$

$v_{FB} = 6$ or -4

Substituting for the velocity of the other cart, it is determined that cart A has a velocity of -4 m/s when cart B has a velocity of 6 m/s and that cart A has a velocity of 6 m/s when cart B has a velocity of -4 m/s. Only one of these combinations is possible. The second combination is not possible, because the carts would have to pass each other—and that is not possible on the track. The original quick and very important solution is proved: When two objects of equal mass collide elastically and head-on (as on a track), they exchange velocities.

138. (A) To conserve both momentum and kinetic energy, the first nickel stops and transfers all its momentum to the second nickel, which moves along a line with the first nickel's velocity. In choice (B), momentum and kinetic energy would be conserved mathematically, but this does not account for the force the first nickel exerts on the stationary nickel. In choice (C), both momentum and kinetic energy could be conserved if the numbers were right, but this wouldn't happen in an elastic, head-on collision of two objects of equal mass. Choice (D) would be the solution if the nickels collided off-center, and not head-on.

139. (A) When the two nickels collide, they exert equal forces on each other but in opposite directions. The force of the second nickel on the first stops the first one, and the equal amount of force of the first nickel on the second causes the second one to start moving with the same momentum that the first nickel had before the collision. The forces are in line with each other in a head-on collision, so the subsequent motion is along a line.

140. (D) By conservation of momentum, the carts move away from each other in opposite directions with the same momentum. Since cart A has twice the mass, it will have half the velocity of cart B and in the opposite direction; thus, cart B has a higher velocity. Regardless of their horizontal velocities, however, the carts start at the same height from the floor, so they will hit the floor at the same time. The time in the air depends only on the height, and not on horizontal speed or the mass of an object.

141. (D) It is necessary to consider components of the velocities in order to conserve linear momentum in the east-west (x) direction and in the north-south (y) direction. The two objects will combine to form one object in a totally inelastic collision, so there is only one 6 kg object moving after the collision. The x component of the new object's momentum is equal to the original momentum in the x direction: (4 kg)(10 m/s), or 40 kg·m/s west. The y component of the new object's momentum is equal to the original momentum in the y direction: (2 kg)(5 m/s), or 10 kg·m/s north. The resultant of these is calculated using the Pythagorean theorem.

$$R = \sqrt{R_x^2 + R_y^2} = \sqrt{10^2 + 40^2} = \sqrt{1700} = 41 \text{ m/s northwest}$$

The actual direction of motion is at an angle that is more west than north, since the west (x) component is much larger: $\tan \theta = (10/40)$ and $\theta = 14°$ north of west.

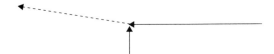

142. (B) First, conservation of momentum is used to determine the final velocity of the 2 kg cart. Then, the kinetic energy of each cart is calculated, both before and after the collision. Finally, the kinetic energies of the two carts before and after the collision are added to determine the change in total kinetic energy during the collision. That change is assumed to be the loss to thermal energy of the surroundings during the collision.

(1) $p_o = p_f$

$m_A v_{oA} + m_B v_{oB} = m_A v_{fA} + m_B v_{fB}$

$(1 \text{ kg})(2 \text{ m/s}) + (2 \text{ kg})(-2 \text{ m/s}) = (1 \text{ kg})(-2 \text{ m/s}) + 0$

(2) $\Delta K = K_f - K_o$

$K_o = \frac{1}{2} m_A v_{oA}^2 + \frac{1}{2} m_B v_{oB}^2 = \frac{1}{2}(1 \text{ kg})(2 \text{ m/s})^2 + \frac{1}{2}(2 \text{ kg})(-2 \text{ m/s})^2 = 6 \text{ J}$

$K_f = \frac{1}{2} m_A v_{fA}^2 + \frac{1}{2} m_B v_{fB}^2 = \frac{1}{2}(1 \text{ kg})(-2 \text{ m/s})^2 + 0 = 2 \text{ J}$

$\Delta K = K_f - K_o = 2 \text{ J} - 6 \text{ J} = -4 \text{ J}$

The negative sign of the answer indicates that kinetic energy is lost from the system, but since the question asked only "how much" loss, the sign is not necessary.

143. (C) First, conservation of momentum is used to determine the final velocity of the combined carts. Then, the kinetic energy of each cart before the collision is calculated, as well as that of the combined carts after the collision. Finally, the kinetic energies of the two carts before the collision and of the combined carts after the collision are added to determine the change in total kinetic energy during the collision. That change is assumed to be the loss to thermal energy of the surroundings during the collision.

(1) $p_o = p_f$

$m_A v_{oA} + m_B v_{oB} = m_A v_{fA} + m_B v_{fB}$

$(1.5 \text{ kg})(2 \text{ m/s}) + (2.0 \text{ kg})(-2 \text{ m/s}) = (1.5 \text{ kg} + 2.0 \text{ kg})v_f$

$v_f = -0.33 \text{ m/s}$

(2) $\Delta K = K_f - K_o$

$K_o = \frac{1}{2} m_A v_{oA}^2 + \frac{1}{2} m_B v_{oB}^2 = \frac{1}{2}(1.5 \text{ kg})(2 \text{ m/s})^2 + \frac{1}{2}(2.0 \text{ kg})(-2 \text{ m/s})^2 = 7.0 \text{ J}$

$K_f = \frac{1}{2}(m_A + m_B)v_{fB}^2 = \frac{1}{2}(3.5 \text{ kg})(-33 \text{ m/s})^2 = 0.6 \text{ J}$

$\Delta K = K_f - K_o = 0.6 \text{ J} - 7.0 \text{ J} = -6.4 \text{ J}$

The negative sign of the answer means that kinetic energy is lost from the system—in this case, most of it. Therefore, the carts are moving very slowly after the collision.

144. (B) A few insights will make what seems like a lengthy problem much simpler. Since the blocks are identical (that is, they have the same mass) and their trajectories are such that the horizontal velocities of the blocks form at right angles, an elastic collision between the two blocks can be assumed. In this special case, both linear momentum and kinetic energy are conserved in the horizontal plane. Neither rolling motion nor friction on the track need to be considered, since the linear velocity of the moving block just before it hits is the objective. (Note, however, that momentum and kinetic energy are not conserved vertically as the blocks fall, since the gravitational force is an intervening external force in that dimension.) The Pythagorean theorem can be used to determine the relationship between the original velocity of the block coming down the track (v_o) and the velocities of the two blocks immediately after the collision. (1) The height of the desk is used to determine the time it takes the blocks to fall to the floor. (2) The horizontal distances, along with this time, are used to determine the velocities. (3) The Pythagorean theorem is used to relate the velocities.

(1) $t = \sqrt{\dfrac{2h}{g}} = \sqrt{\dfrac{2(1 \text{ m})}{9.8 \text{ m/s}^2}} = 0.45 \text{ s}$

(2) $v_1 = \dfrac{d_1}{t} = \dfrac{0.5 \text{ m}}{0.45 \text{ s}} = 1.1 \text{ m/s}$

$v_2 = \dfrac{d_2}{t} = \dfrac{0.25 \text{ m}}{0.45 \text{ s}} = 0.55 \text{ m/s}$

(3) $v_o^2 = (1.1 \text{ m/s})^2 + (0.55 \text{ m/s})^2$

$v_o = 1.2 \text{ m/s}$

The solution may seem math-intensive, but it helps to realize that it takes an object about ½ s to fall one meter from rest near Earth's surface; this fact can be used to calculate the velocities of the blocks after the collision. Additionally, the Pythagorean calculation can be estimated; since the sum of the squares of the velocities is just a little over 1, the square root is closer to 1 than to choices (A), (C), and (D).

145. (D) Since the track is level at the point of collision and there are no external forces, such as friction or gravitational force, applied to the system, linear momentum is conserved in the horizontal plane. Once the blocks collide and begin to fall, however, the gravitational force is an external force that changes both momentum and kinetic energy. Choice (A) cannot be true, because kinetic energy is not conserved as the blocks fall; instead, gravitational potential energy is converted to additional kinetic energy. Choice (B) cannot be true, because the gravitational force increases both momentum and kinetic energy as the blocks fall. Choice (C) cannot be true, because the gravitational force exerted on the blocks as they fall increases their momentum, and therefore linear momentum is not conserved in that vertical direction, or third dimension.

146. (D) Since each velocity vector is the same, the momentum vector for each piece will equal its mass times its velocity; thus, each momentum vector is longer by a factor of the mass. For example, the momentum vector for the 3 g piece is three times the size of the momentum vector for the 1 g piece. Since the explosion takes place on a level table, the gravitational force is not in the plane of the table, and so momentum is conserved in the plane of the table. Momentum must be considered in each direction on the plane. The components in the left-right direction are considered separately from the components in the up-down direction. Choice (A) cannot be correct, because the momentum of the 3 g piece in the up direction is not balanced in the down direction, and therefore momentum is not conserved. Choice (B) cannot be correct, because the momentum of the 1 g piece in the up direction will be far less than the momentum of the 3 g piece in the down direction. Choice (C) cannot be correct, because the momentum of the 1 g piece to the left will be far less than the sum of the momenta of the other two pieces to the right. Choice (D) is possible, because the momentum in the up-down direction could add to zero, and the momentum in the left-right direction could add to zero.

Chapter 5: Torque and Equilibrium

147. (C) The net force on an object is zero if there is no acceleration in any dimension. In choice (A), the box sliding down a frictionless ramp must be accelerating, since there is no friction force on the box to oppose the component of the gravitational force accelerating the box down the ramp. In choice (B), there must be an unbalanced centripetal force to keep the satellite in a circular path. In choice (C), the box is sliding at constant speed, so the net force horizontally must be zero. In choice (D), the hammer must be accelerating, since there is no atmosphere on the moon to provide a drag force to keep the hammer from accelerating under the influence of gravity.

148. (A) The problem is set up so that the horizontal components of the tensions in all three wires add—as vectors—to zero. This creates a horizontal equilibrium to keep the post in an upright position. The horizontal component for each tension is equal to $T \cos 60°$. Since the first two vectors have horizontal components that are perpendicular to each other (east and north), the Pythagorean theorem can be used to determine the resultant. The third vector required to balance will have a horizontal component that is equal in magnitude to the resultant but in the opposite direction; it is called the "equilibrant." Choice (A) correctly uses the horizontal components to determine the magnitude of the tension in the equilibrant.

149. (C) The friction force of the ramp on the box is equal in magnitude to the component of the gravitational force that is parallel to the ramp, which is $10 \sin 30°$. Since the box is sliding at constant speed, the net force exerted on the box in the direction of motion must be zero.

150. (B) Since the ladder is in static equilibrium, the net force in each direction is equal to zero. Therefore, the normal force of the floor on the ladder and the weight of the ladder are equal. The friction force of the floor on the ladder is equal to the normal force of the wall on the ladder. In addition, the friction force is equal to the coefficient of friction times the normal force of the floor on the ladder. Since the coefficient is less than one, the friction force must be less than the normal force.

151. (B) As an object oscillates on a spring, it is in equilibrium at the position where the forces are in balance, that is, where velocity is maximum, acceleration is zero, and displacement is zero.

152. (B) As the Ping-Pong ball accelerates due to the gravitational force exerted on it, the air drag force upward on the ball increases. (Drag forces increase with the speed of an object moving through a fluid.) At terminal velocity, the air drag force is equal to the weight of the ball and the ball is in equilibrium. At that point, the acceleration of the ball is zero and the ball subsequently falls at constant speed, which is called terminal velocity.

153. (D) The pendulum is in equilibrium in the horizontal direction, because there are no forces in the x direction at the bottom of the motion, assuming air friction is negligible. This does not, however, allow choice (B) to be correct, since there is no accelerating force at the bottom; the pendulum continues to move at that point due to the inertia of the pendulum bob. In addition, the pendulum is in equilibrium in the vertical direction at the bottom of its swing, since the tension upward must be equal to the weight of the pendulum bob plus enough force to provide the centripetal force to keep the pendulum moving in a circular path.

154. (C) This is an equilibrium situation. For the sled to slide at constant speed down the hill, the net force on the sled must be zero. Choice (A) is not correct, because inertia is not a force. Choice (B) is not correct, because there is a force propelling the sled down the hill—the component of the gravitational force that is parallel to the hill. Choice (D) is not correct, because for the sled to be in equilibrium and move at constant speed, a friction force must be present in the opposite direction of the gravitational force component directed down the hill.

155. (D) The force shown will cause the wheel to rotate clockwise, so the friction torque must be counterclockwise to create balanced torques and an equilibrium situation for the wheel to rotate at constant speed. The clockwise torque will be calculated using $\tau = R_\perp F$ $= (.20 \text{ m})(100 \text{ N}) = 20 \text{ N·m}$. The counterclockwise torque must also be equal to 20 N·m. The axle radius is one fourth as much, so the friction force must be 4 times greater than the applied force, or 400 N. However, the question asks for torque, not force, so the friction torque is 400 N × 0.05 m, or 20 N·m counterclockwise.

156. **(C)** Actually, the system will still balance if the center of mass of the system of sticks is anywhere to the left of the edge of the table, so that gravitational force on that center of mass cannot exert a torque to cause the sticks to fall. The center of mass of the system can be determined by taking the edge of the table as a pivot, or zero point. Since all the sticks have the same mass, the distance of the center of mass of each stick from the edge of the table is multiplied by the stick's mass to find the torque due to the gravitational force on that stick. Any value to the left of the table edge is considered negative. All four values are then added. If the result is zero, the center of mass of the system of sticks is above the pivot, so there is no net torque to cause the sticks to fall. If the result is negative, the center of mass of the system is over the table, so the system will balance. In addition, each stick must have its center of mass above the object below it. Choice (B) could work, but it does not meet the condition that the top stick is entirely beyond the table edge.

157. **(B)** As the wheels roll, they are moving backward at the instant they touch the pavement, so the friction force from the pavement on the tires is forward. The friction force is the force that moves the car forward in the same way that the friction force from the floor is forward on your feet as you take a step—and that friction force causes you to move forward.

158. **(D)** The torque that you exert is your force, F, times the radius of the steering wheel. For the car, the torque is $30F$, and for the truck it is $40F$. The increase is $10F$, and the percent increase is the amount of increase divided by the original.

$$\% \text{ increase} = \frac{\text{increase}}{\text{original}} = \frac{10F}{30F} = 33\%$$

This increase in torque using the same applied force makes it easier to drive the much larger truck.

159. **(D)** Using the edge of the roof as the pivot, the clockwise torque exerted by the acrobat on the board cannot be more than the counterclockwise torque exerted by the weight of the board applied at its center of mass at the center of the board. The clockwise torque exerted by the acrobat (force times distance to the pivot) is $(60 \text{ kg})(9.8 \text{ m/s}^2)(x)$. The counterclockwise torque exerted by the board is $(20 \text{ kg})(9.8 \text{ m/s}^2)(2 \text{ ft})$. (Note: One third of the length of the board, or 4 ft, extends over the edge, so the center of the board is 6 ft from the end and 2 ft from the edge of the building.) Therefore, $60x = 40$ and $x = \frac{2}{3}$ ft, or 8 inches.

160. **(B)** Torque is force applied (in this case, the weight of the rider) times the distance from the downward applied force to the axle, measured horizontally: $\tau = (50 \text{ kg})(9.8 \text{ m/s}^2)$ $(0.18 \text{ m}) = $ about $(50)(10)(0.2) = 100$ N·m. Of course, the torque applied by the rider changes as the pedal goes around in a circle. The maximum torque is applied when the pedal is farthest forward and moving downward; the average torque for any complete circle is probably close to half of that value.

161. (B) To lift the weight slowly, the clockwise torque exerted by the object must be equal to the counterclockwise torque exerted by the lower arm.

$\tau = R_\perp F = (0.3 \text{ m})(9.8 \text{ m/s}^2)(5 \text{ kg}) = 15 \text{ N·m}$

162. (A) Torque is equal to force (in this case, the weight of the object) times the distance from the line of force to the pivot. The clockwise torque is due to the weight of the rod and the weight of the smaller object.

$\tau = R_\wedge F = (0.7 \text{ m})(9.8 \text{ m/s}^2)(0.5 \text{ kg}) + (0.2 \text{ m})(9.8 \text{ m/s}^2)(0.2 \text{ kg}) = 3.9 \text{ N·m}$

The counterclockwise torque is due to the weight of the larger object.

$\tau = R_\wedge F = (0.3 \text{ m})(9.8 \text{ m/s}^2)(1.0 \text{ kg}) = 3.0 \text{ N·m}$

The net torque is 0.9 N·m clockwise.

163. (D) For a condition of equilibrium, the object or system may be either stationary or moving at constant speed—as long as acceleration is zero. The net torque and net force in every dimension must be zero.

164. (A) Forces C and D exert clockwise torques, and forces A and B exert counterclockwise torques. Torque is the product of force and radius in each case, since the forces are all tangential, making them perpendicular to the radius. For present purposes, clockwise torques are positive and counterclockwise torques are negative.

Torque A $= (20 \text{ N})(0.10 \text{ m}) = -2 \text{ N·m}$
Torque B $= (50 \text{ N})(0.02 \text{ m}) = -1 \text{ N·m}$
Torque C $= (30 \text{ N})(0.10 \text{ m}) = 3 \text{ N·m}$
Torque D $= (10 \text{ N})(0.10 \text{ m}) = 1 \text{ N·m}$
Net torque $= 1$ N·m clockwise

165. (A) Torque is equal to the applied force times the perpendicular distance to the axis of rotation. Since each of the four torques is along a tangent (and the tangent is always perpendicular to the radius), in each case the force is multiplied by the radius at the point $\tau = R_\perp F$. For present purposes, clockwise torques are positive and counterclockwise torques are negative. The net torque is the sum of the four individual torques.

$\Sigma\tau = (10 \text{ N})(0.3 \text{ m}) + (30 \text{ N})(0.3 \text{ m}) - (50 \text{ N})(0.1 \text{ m}) - (20 \text{ N})(0.3 \text{ m}) = 1.0 \text{ N·m}$
$\Sigma\tau = I\alpha$
$1.0 \text{ N·m} = (4.0 \text{ kg·m}^2)(\alpha)$
$\alpha = 0.25 \text{ rad/s}^2$

166. **(D)** For the system to balance (that is, maintain rotational equilibrium), the net torque at the fulcrum must be zero. In other words, the net clockwise torque on the rod must be equal in magnitude to the net counterclockwise torque. Without the added 1 kg mass, the clockwise torque ($\tau = R_{\perp}F$) is $mgR = $ (2 kg)(9.8 m/s²)(⅔L). The counterclockwise torque is $mgR = $ (6 kg)(9.8 m/s²)(⅓L). The net torque clockwise is $4mgL/3$, and the counterclockwise torque is $6mgL/3$. To balance, $2mgL/3$ must be added to the right side, recognizing that $m = 1$ kg.

$$\frac{2mgL}{3} = mgR$$

$$\frac{2L}{3} = R$$

Therefore, the extra 1 kg mass needs to be attached $2L/3$ from the pivot, meaning it will be attached to the right end of the rod.

167. **(D)** A diagram is made, showing the forces being exerted on the bridge. (1) The net force in the y direction (vertically) must be zero, so the two piers together must support the entire weight of the bridge plus car, or $W = mg = $ (22,000 kg)(10 m/s²) = 220,000 N. (2) A fulcrum is then positioned at one end (in this case, the left end) and the clockwise and counterclockwise torques are set equal, since the net torque on the bridge about any axis must be zero.

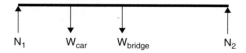

(1) $\Sigma F_y = 0$

$N_1 + N_2 - W_{car} - W_{bridge} = 0$

$N_1 + N_2 = $ (22,000 kg)(9.8 m/s²) = 220,000 N

(2) $\tau_{cw} = \tau_{ccw}$

$(W_{car})(5 \text{ m}) + (W_{bridge})(10 \text{ m}) = N_2(20 \text{ m})$

$(20,000 \text{ N})(5 \text{ m}) + (200,000 \text{ N})(10 \text{ m}) = N_2(20 \text{ m})$

$N_2 = 105,000$ N

$N_1 = 220,000$ N $- 105,000$ N $= 115,000$ N

168. **(D)** Balanced torques are used to solve for the unknown mass of the meter stick.

$\Sigma \tau = 0$

$\tau_{cw} = \tau_{ccw}$

(0.35 kg)(9.8 m/s²)(0.35 m) + (m_{stick})(9.8 m/s²)(0.15 m) = (0.80 kg)(9.8 m/s²)(0.2 m)

$m = 0.25$ kg

169. (B) The net force in each direction must be equal to zero, and the net torque on the meter stick must be equal to zero. This problem becomes easier by recognizing the $1\text{-}2\text{-}\sqrt{3}$ right-triangle relationship, since the length of the meter stick and the distance of the meter stick from the wall at the base are in a 1:2 ratio.

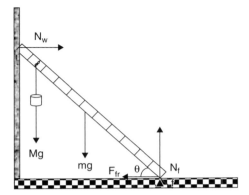

$\Sigma F_x = 0$, and therefore $N_{wall} = F_{f, \, floor}$

$\Sigma F_y = 0$, and therefore $N_{floor} = W_{meter \, stick} + W_{hanging \, mass}$

A pivot is set where the meter stick meets the floor, and the clockwise and counterclockwise torques are set equal.

$\tau_{cw} = \tau_{ccw}$

$(N_{wall})(\sqrt{3}/2 \text{ m}) = (W_{meter \, stick})(0.25 \text{ m}) + (W_{hanging \, mass})(0.375 \text{ m})$

$(N_{wall})(\sqrt{3}/2 \text{ m}) = (0.5 \text{ kg})(9.8 \text{ m/s}^2)(0.25 \text{ m}) + (1 \text{ kg})(9.8 \text{ m/s}^2)(0.375 \text{ m})$

$N_{wall} = F_{f, \, floor} = 5.7 \text{ N}$

Note: In each torque term, the force is multiplied by the perpendicular distance from the line of force to the pivot in order to determine the torque.

170. (B) The clockwise torque exerted by the person's downward force is equal (at a minimum) to the counterclockwise torque exerted by the lid of the can. Setting the torques equal:

$\tau_{cw} = \tau_{ccw}$

$F_{person}(0.11 \text{ m}) = F_{lid}(0.01 \text{ m})$

$(100 \text{ N})(0.11 \text{ m}) = F_{lid}(0.01 \text{ m})$

$F_{lid} = 1{,}100 \text{ N}$

171. (B) If the pivot is set at the point of connection of the beam to the wall, then the sum of clockwise torques must be equal to the sum of counterclockwise torques. By setting the pivot at this point, the force from the wall exerts no torque, since the line of force runs through the pivot.

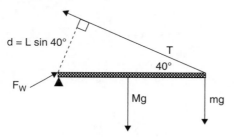

Choice (B) correctly shows each force applied to the beam multiplied by its lever arm (the perpendicular distance from the line of force to the pivot). Choices (A) and (D) ignore the force applied by the hinge between the beam and the wall in accounting for horizontal and vertical forces. Choice (C) uses the incorrect component to determine the lever arm for the tension.

172. (D) For the ladder to remain stable, the net force in each direction must be equal to zero. The only vertical forces are the weight of the ladder downward and the normal force from the floor upward, so they must be equal: $Mg = N_{floor}$. The only horizontal forces are the normal force from the wall to the right and the friction force of the floor on the ladder to the left, so they must be equal: $N_{wall} = F_{floor}$.

Since only the mass of the ladder is given, torque must be used to solve the problem. The pivot is set at the point where the ladder touches the floor, and clockwise and counterclockwise torques are set equal to each other. This problem becomes easier by recognizing the 1-2-$\sqrt{3}$ right-triangle relationship, since the length of the ladder and the distance of the ladder from the wall at the base are in a 1:2 ratio. Therefore, the height of the ladder on the wall is $\sqrt{3}$ m.

$$\tau_{cw} = \tau_{ccw}$$

$$(N_{wall})(\sqrt{3} \text{ m}) = (m_{ladder})(g)(0.5 \text{ m})$$

$$N_{wall} = F_f = \frac{(6 \text{ kg})(9.8 \text{ m/s}^2)(0.5 \text{ m})}{\sqrt{3}} = 17 \text{ N}$$

173. (B) If the meter stick and the unknown object balance when the pivot is at the 60 cm mark, then the clockwise and counterclockwise torques exerted by the weight of the meter stick on one side and the unknown object on the other side of the pivot must be equal. Each torque is equal to the weight of the object times its distance from the pivot. The torque due to the meter stick's weight is mgR, or $(0.1 \text{ kg})(9.8 \text{ m/s}^2)(0.10 \text{ m}) = 0.10 \text{ N·m}$. The torque due to the weight of the unknown object is mgR, or $m(9.8 \text{ m/s}^2)(0.2 \text{ m})$. Since the force due to the unknown object is twice as far from the pivot, and the torques are equal, then the mass of the unknown object must be half as much as the mass of the stick, or 50 g.

174. (D) On the bottom branch, the rectangle on the right exerts a torque of (0.1 kg) $(9.8 \text{ m/s}^2)(0.1 \text{ m}) = 1 \text{ N·m}$, so the torque on the left also must be 1 N·m. The weight of the stick exerts a torque of $(0.01 \text{ kg})(9.8 \text{ m/s}^2)(0.1 \text{ m}) = 0.01 \text{ N·m}$, and the triangle exerts a torque of $(0.33 \text{ kg})(9.8 \text{ m/s}^2)(0.3 \text{ m}) = 0.99 \text{ N·m}$—for a total of 1 N·m. Now, the entire weight of the bottom branch, which is $(0.133 \text{ kg})(9.8 \text{ m/s}^2) = 1.33 \text{ N}$, is used to determine torque in the top branch.

The torque on the right side of the connection is due to the weight of the bottom branch, which is $(1.33 \text{ N})(0.3 \text{ m})$, or about 3.99 N·m. The torque on the right side due to the weight of the stick is $(0.01 \text{ kg})(9.8 \text{ m/s}^2)(0.1 \text{ m}) = 0.01 \text{ N·m}$. The total torque on the right, therefore, is 4 N·m. Consequently, the torque on the left must also be 4 N·m. The calculation is $m(9.8 \text{ m/s}^2)(0.1 \text{ m}) = 4 \text{ N·m}$, and $m = 4 \text{ kg}$.

175. (D) For the rod to balance, the torque exerted by the objects on each side of the pivot must balance. The equation to calculate torque is $\tau = RF$, where R is the distance from the attachment of the object to the pivot and F is the weight of the attached object. The distance R must be measured perpendicular to the force F, but in this case, the rod will be horizontal when balanced, so the forces will all be vertical—and perpendicular to the measured distances. To balance the torques on each side of the pivot, the force is equal to mg, but each term will have g in it, so g is canceled in every term and only mass times distance must be examined on each side of the pivot. In choice (A), the sum of the torques on the right side is $(1)(1.0) + (2)(0.5)$, or 2.0, and the torque on the left side is $(3)(0.5)$, or 1.5—which doesn't balance. In choice (B), the sum of the torques on the right side is $(1)(1.0) + (2)(0.5)$, or 2.0, and the torque on the left side is $(3)(2.0)$, or 6.0—which doesn't balance. In choice (C), the sum of the torques on the right side is $(1)(2.0) + (2)(1.0)$, or 4.0, and the torque on the left side is $(3)(0.5)$, or 1.5—which doesn't balance. In choice (D), the sum of the torques on the right side is $(1)(2.0) + (2)(2.0)$, or 6.0, which equals the torque on the left side: $(3)(2.0)$, or 6.0.

Chapter 6: Work, Energy, and Power

176. (C) Kinetic energy is equal to $\frac{1}{2}mv^2$. Since the object is accelerating as it falls, its velocity at any point after it is dropped can be determined using the following formula.

$$v_f^2 = v_o^2 + 2ad$$

The acceleration, a, is equal to g and the initial velocity is zero, since the object has been dropped from rest. Doubling the distance the object has fallen also doubles the square of the velocity. Since kinetic energy depends on the square of velocity, we conclude that doubling the distance also doubles the kinetic energy.

This result can also be determined by the principles of energy conservation. When the object is dropped, it has gravitational potential energy. Halfway to the ground, the object has half as much potential energy as it had when it was dropped—and half as much kinetic energy as it will have when it hits the ground.

177. (D) The loss in gravitational energy of the pendulum bob (relative to Earth) is equal to the gain in kinetic energy of the bob as it passes through equilibrium.

$$mg\Delta h = \frac{1}{2}m(\Delta v)^2$$
$$v = \sqrt{2gh} = \sqrt{(2)(9.8 \text{ m/s}^2)(0.2)} = \sqrt{4} = 2 \text{ m/s}$$

178. (C) The space vehicle moves more slowly in its orbit when it is farther from Earth. As the vehicle moves farther away, the gravitational force of Earth on the vehicle is less, and this provides the centripetal force to keep the object in orbit. Therefore, if the centripetal force is less, the speed of the vehicle is less.

$$F_G = F_C = \frac{mv^2}{R}$$

When the speed is less, the kinetic energy is less.

179. (B) The kinetic energy of the rock when it hits the ground will be the total of the original kinetic energy and the kinetic energy converted from gravitational potential energy during the fall.

$$K_{total} = K_o + \Delta U = \frac{1}{2}mv^2 + mgh = \frac{1}{2}(0.5 \text{ kg})(5.0 \text{ m/s})^2 + (0.5 \text{ kg})(9.8 \text{ m/s}^2)(20 \text{ m})$$
$$= 106.25 \text{ J}$$

180. (D) Kinetic energy is $\frac{1}{2}mv^2$, so change in kinetic energy (ΔK) is final K minus original K. The amount of time this takes is not a factor.

$$\Delta K = K_f - K_o = \frac{1}{2}mv_f^2 - \frac{1}{2}mv_o^2 = \frac{1}{2}(2{,}000 \text{ kg})[(20 \text{ m/s})^2 - (10 \text{ m/s})^2] = 300{,}000 \text{ J}$$

181. (B) This question involves the concept that energy can be measured in electron volts as well as in joules. One electron volt is equal to 1.6×10^{-19} J, since one electron volt is the amount of energy gained by one electron moving through an electric potential difference of one volt. The answer is the product of the number of electrons and the electric potential difference: $\Delta K = qV = (1 \text{ e}^-)(12 \text{ V}) = 12 \text{ eV}$.

182. (D) Joules, ergs, and electron volts are all units of work or energy. The watt is a unit of power, or energy divided by time.

183. (B) The object has an initial kinetic energy due to its horizontal motion at the moment it starts falling. Therefore, choices (C) and (D) are not possible, because they start at zero when time is zero. The relationship between kinetic energy and time is a curve, since $K = \frac{1}{2}mv^2$, and the kinetic energy increases as the object falls.

184. (D) Due to conservation of energy, the total energy of the block as it slides off the roof is the sum of its potential and kinetic energies. At the ground, all the mechanical energy is kinetic energy, so the kinetic energy just before the block hits the ground is equal to the total mechanical energy at the top, just before the fall.

$$E = mgh + \frac{1}{2}mv^2 = (2 \text{ kg})(10 \text{ m/s}^2)(4 \text{ m}) + \frac{1}{2}(2 \text{ kg})(3 \text{ m/s})^2 = 89 \text{ J}$$

185. (C) The gravitational potential energy, mgh, is equal to 80 J. Just before the ball hits the floor, this gravitational potential energy is converted to 80 J of kinetic energy. Then, 10% of this, or 8 J, is converted to thermal energy during the collision with the floor, leaving 72 J of kinetic energy as the ball rebounds.

186. (A) The object has an initial kinetic energy due to its horizontal motion at the moment it starts falling, then adds kinetic energy as it falls. However, the largest height is at the right on the x axis, so as the object falls, the kinetic energy is determined by moving left on the x axis. At height zero—just before the object lands—the object has the highest kinetic energy. The relationship between height and kinetic energy is linear, since kinetic energy increases as potential energy decreases: $mgh = \frac{1}{2}mv^2 = K$. In choices (B), (C), and (D), kinetic energy increases with the height, which does not happen as the object falls.

187. (D) Assuming no loss of energy due to air friction, mechanical energy is conserved. The kinetic energy just before the rock hits the ground is equal to the total energy as the rock leaves the top of the building. The total energy at the top is kinetic energy plus gravitational potential energy.

188. (C) If the larger object moves downward 0.1 m, the smaller object must move upward the same amount. The change in gravitational potential energy of the smaller object is equal to mgh: $(0.02 \text{ kg})(9.8 \text{ m/s}^2)(0.1 \text{ m}) = 0.02 \text{ J}$.

189. (B) Moving the object to a position two Earth radii above the surface means the new distance between the center of the object and the center of Earth has been tripled. The equation $U = mgh$ is only an approximation for gravitational potential energy when an object is located on the surface—and gives no real sense that a single object can't have potential energy.

Gravitational potential energy is a property of a system of objects and depends on the masses and relative positions of the objects. By examining the equation to determine the gravitational potential energy for two objects of masses M and m, it is apparent that tripling the distance between the objects will make the new value of U equal to one third of its original value. Therefore, the ratio of the magnitude of the original potential energy to the potential energy at the greater distance is 3:1.

$$U_G = \frac{-GMm}{R}$$

However, it should be noted, in examining this equation, that the gravitational potential energy has a negative sign. The larger negative value for potential energy on the surface is actually a *smaller* number, as might be expected. Moving an object three times as far from the Earth's center produces a gravitational potential energy of the Earth-object system that is a *smaller negative* number—which is actually larger, as might be predicted. For example, a moving satellite must have less kinetic energy (and move more slowly) as its orbit is changed to a greater distance from Earth, since the total energy must be constant. Increasing the potential energy (a smaller negative number) decreases the kinetic energy of the Earth-satellite system.

190. (C) As Earth orbits the sun, the total mechanical energy of the Earth-sun system must remain constant. At the point in Earth's elliptical orbit when it moves closer to the sun, Earth moves faster and has greater kinetic energy. Therefore, the gravitational potential energy of the Earth-sun system decreases.

191. (D) The gravitational potential energy, U, of the original system is calculated by using the following equation.

$$U_1 = \frac{-GMm}{R}$$

The potential energy of the second system is calculated by doubling each mass and halving the distance between the particles.

$$U_2 = \frac{-G(2M)(2m)}{\frac{1}{2}R} = 8U_1$$

192. (C) Spring potential energy is equal to $\frac{1}{2}kx^2$, where x is spring extension. If x is doubled, the potential energy is four times as much, since the spring extension is squared.

193. (D) When the ruler is flexed, it behaves like a spring and has elastic potential energy. Then, when the ruler is released with the rock against it, the potential energy stored in the rock-ruler system is converted to kinetic energy of the rock. When the ruler reaches its equilibrium position, it releases the rock, and the rock moves away with kinetic energy. The mass and velocity of the rock are used to determine its kinetic energy. The elastic potential energy of the ruler is set equal to the kinetic energy of the rock to determine the elastic constant, k.

$$\Delta U = \Delta K$$

$$\frac{1}{2}kx^2 = \frac{1}{2}mv^2$$

$$k = \frac{mv^2}{x^2} = \frac{(0.1 \text{ kg})(2.0 \text{ m/s})^2}{(0.05 \text{ m})^2} = 160 \text{ N/m}$$

194. (B) Spring potential energy is dependent on amplitude: $U = \frac{1}{2}kx^2$. Amplitude is greatest at the peaks on the graph, whether positive or negative, because spring displacement, x, is greatest. At all other times, the displacement of the spring is zero, so the spring potential energy is zero.

195. (D) The spring equation is in the form $x(t) = A \cos \omega t$, where $\omega = 10$ and $m = 2$ kg.

$$\omega = \sqrt{\frac{k}{m}}$$

$$10 = \sqrt{\frac{k}{2}}$$

$$k = 200 \text{ N/m}$$

196. (D) Using conservation of energy, the potential energy of the ball-spring system is converted to kinetic energy in the ball: $\frac{1}{2}kx^2 = \frac{1}{2}mv^2$. Substituting mass ($m = 0.1$ kg), speed ($v = 10$ m/s), and displacement ($x = 0.1$ m), the spring constant, k, is calculated as 1,000 N/m.

197. (C) The friction force is nonconservative, since work done by the friction force is converted to thermal energy of molecules in the object's environment, thereby reducing the total amount of mechanical energy. When calculating work done by friction, the conversion to thermal energy takes place during the entire contact time between objects, so the entire path taken must be used in calculation. The gravitational force is a conservative force; work done by the gravitational force conserves mechanical energy and does not depend on the path taken by the object.

198. (C) The friction force is a nonconservative force, since it does negative work on the ball, thereby reducing the total amount of mechanical energy.

199. (C) The work done by the gravitational force is equal to the weight of the object (mg) times the vertical distance the object slides (10 m). Since the gravitational force is a conservative force, the path length, or total distance that the object travels, is irrelevant. The gravitational force on the object is directed downward at all times during the object's trip down the hill, and the direction of displacement of the object is downward, so the product (or dot product) is positive.

Another approach to the problem uses the work-energy theorem, where the work done by gravity is equal to the increase in kinetic energy. If the decrease in gravitational potential energy is used to calculate the kinetic energy, the work is equal to mgh: $\Delta U = W = mg\Delta h = (2 \text{ kg})(9.8 \text{ m/s}^2)(10 \text{ m}) = 196 \text{ J}$.

200. (B) Work done on the spring is equal to the applied force, F, multiplied by the displacement of the spring, x: $W = Fx$. The force is not a constant force; it requires more force to stretch a spring each unit of distance as the spring is stretched further from equilibrium. The average force from the data in the graph is one half times the maximum force, or one half of 100 N. Therefore, the work is 50 N × 2 m, or 100 J.

Another approach to the problem is to use the area under the line—a triangle—to calculate the work done (which would also be the potential energy of the spring system when stretched this distance). The area of the triangle is $A = \frac{1}{2}bh$, or $\frac{1}{2}(2 \text{ m})(100 \text{ N})$.

201. (D) Work is defined as force times displacement, with the force and displacement in the same direction ($W = F \cdot s$). Since the velocity vector of the car at any moment is on a tangent to the circle, the displacement vector is also a tangent. By definition, centripetal force is inward, toward the center, along a radius—and the radius is always perpendicular to a tangent. Since there is no component of force in the direction of displacement, the product is zero and the work is zero.

Another approach to the problem uses the work-energy theorem, where the work done is equal to the change in kinetic energy. Since the track is level and the car's speed is constant, neither the kinetic energy nor the potential energy of the car changes during its motion. If there is no change in energy, work is zero.

202. (B) First, the work done by friction is negative, since it is in the opposite direction of the motion of the box. Work is defined as the product of force and displacement, using components of both that are along the same dimension: $W = F \cdot s = Fs \cos \theta$. Since both the friction force and the displacement of the box are parallel to the floor, the work is the product of the friction force and the distance, d. By definition, the friction force is equal to the coefficient of friction times the normal force—and the normal force is equal to the weight of the box (mg) on a level surface.

$$W = -(F_f)(d) = -(\mu N)(d) = -\mu mgd$$

203. (A) The work done by the force on the box is calculated as $W = F \cdot s = Fs \cos \theta$. To calculate work, components of force and displacement must be along the same line. In choice (A), the force and displacement are both parallel to the floor, so the maximum work is done by F in this case. In the other three choices, only a component of the force F is parallel to the floor, and since the component is always less than F, the work done in each of those cases is less.

204. (A) The friction force between the car's tires and the roadway is the only force in the right direction (toward the center of the circle in which the car is turning) to provide the centripetal force. Since the car is on a level road and the friction force is equal to the coefficient of friction (μ) times the normal force (and the normal force of the road on the car is equal to the weight of the car), the centripetal force is set equal to μmg. (Note that the mass of the car cancels.)

$$F_{fr} = F_{cent}$$
$$F_{fr} = \mu N = \mu mg$$
$$\therefore \mu mg = \frac{mv^2}{r}$$
$$\mu = \frac{v^2}{gr} = \frac{(10 \text{ m/s})^2}{(10 \text{ m/s}^2)(100 \text{ m})} = 0.1$$

205. (C) The work done by the target in stopping the arrow is equal to the loss in kinetic energy of the arrow. The kinetic energy is $\frac{1}{2}mv^2$, so the work equals $\frac{1}{2}(0.25 \text{ kg})(10 \text{ m/s})^2$, or 12.5 J. The work is force times distance, so the force can be determined by dividing the work by the distance: $W/d = F = 12.5 \text{ J}/0.04 \text{ m} = 312 \text{ N}$. The force of the arrow on the target is equal in magnitude to the force of the target on the arrow.

206. (D) As the ball leaves the top of the platform, its total energy is the sum of its kinetic energy and its gravitational potential energy. The easiest way to solve this problem is to use conservation of mechanical energy. As the ball hits the ground, its total mechanical energy is the same as when it left the platform, except it is now all in the form of kinetic energy.

$$K_{top} + U_{top} = K_{bottom}$$
$$\frac{1}{2}mv_{top}^2 + mgh_{top} = \frac{1}{2}mv_{bottom}^2$$
$$\frac{1}{2}(4.0 \text{ m/s})^2 + (9.8 \text{ m/s}^2)(10 \text{ m}) = \frac{1}{2}v_{bottom}^2$$

The mass is canceled in every term, since the mass of the object does not affect the result. The velocity of the ball when it hits the ground is $v = 15 \text{ m/s}$.

207. (C) The friction force of the floor on the box does work in stopping the box. By the work-energy theorem, the work is equal to the loss in kinetic energy. The coefficient of friction can be estimated from the data given. (Note that the mass of the box cancels, so changing the contents of the box to change the mass of the box would not affect the outcome.)

$W_{fr} = \Delta K$

$F_{fr}d = \frac{1}{2}mv^2$

$(\mu N)d = \frac{1}{2}mv^2$

$(\mu mg)d = \frac{1}{2}mv^2$

$\mu(9.8 \text{ m/s}^2)(1 \text{ m}) = \frac{1}{2}(2 \text{ m/s})^2$

μ is approximately 0.2.

208. (C) The boxes will travel the same distance across the floor. If the boxes are identical otherwise, their masses cancel. It is the work done by the friction force of the floor on each box that stops the box. The work done by friction (which is negative) is set equal to the change in kinetic energy of the box (which is also negative).

$W_{fr} = \Delta K$

$F_{fr}d = \frac{1}{2}mv^2$

$(\mu N)d = \frac{1}{2}mv^2$

$(\mu mg)d = \frac{1}{2}mv^2$

$d = \dfrac{v^2}{2g\mu}$

As long as the boxes are moving at the same speed when they reach the floor and the coefficient of friction between each box and the floor is the same, they will move the same distance before coming to a stop. Mass is not a factor.

209. (C) The maximum net work is done during the time interval when the net change in kinetic energy is greatest. In choice (A), the oscillating object moves from a position where spring potential energy is maximum and kinetic energy is zero to another position where potential energy is maximum. Therefore, the change in kinetic energy ($K_f - K_o$) is zero and work is zero. In choice (B), the oscillating object moves from a position of zero kinetic energy to another position of zero kinetic energy, so the net work is zero. In choice (D), the initial and final positions are at maximum amplitude, where kinetic energy is zero, so no net work is done on the object during this interval. In choice (C), the spring force moves the object from amplitude (where $K = 0$) to equilibrium (where K is maximum), so the maximum amount of net work is done by the spring on the object during this interval.

210. (C) The block loses contact with the spring at the equilibrium, or relaxed, position of the spring, so the block has moved a distance of 5 cm (0.05 m) when it loses contact. The kinetic energy of the block at that point is equal to the spring potential energy of the spring-block system prior to release of the block minus the work done against friction in moving the block across the surface. The work done against friction is equal to the friction force times the distance the block moves to equilibrium, and the friction force is equal to the coefficient of friction times the normal force. The normal force on this level surface is equal to the block's weight, mg.

$U_{\text{spring-block}} = K_{\text{block}} + W_f$

$\frac{1}{2}kx^2 = \frac{1}{2}mv^2 + \mu mg$

$\frac{1}{2}(200 \text{ N/m})(0.05 \text{ m})^2 = \frac{1}{2}(0.5 \text{ kg})(v^2) + (0.02)(0.5 \text{ kg})(9.8\text{m/s}^2)$

$v = 0.1 \text{ m/s}$

211. (C) The potential energy of the spring-putty system when the toy is pushed down is equal to the gravitational potential energy of the system when it reaches its maximum height.

$\Delta U_{\text{spring}} = \Delta U_G$

$\frac{1}{2}kx^2 = mgh$

$\frac{1}{2}k(0.01 \text{ m})^2 = (0.02 \text{ kg})(9.8 \text{ m/s}^2)(0.08 \text{ m})$

$k = 320 \text{ N/m}$

212. (D) The best choice is (D), because the satellite already has some gravitational potential energy with reference to the center of Earth when it is on the surface. (Actually, the Earth-satellite system has gravitational potential energy.) The satellite on the surface also has kinetic energy, since it is moving in a circular path with Earth's surface. The work required to place the satellite in orbit is equal to the sum of the changes in kinetic and potential energies. Choices (A) and (C) are easily eliminated, because their answers involve adding force to energy.

213. (B) In choice (A), the speed doesn't change, so no work is done to increase kinetic or potential energy. However, there is work done against friction (the friction force (μmg) times the distance moved: $W = \mu mgd = (0.05)(20 \text{ kg})(10 \text{ N})(10 \text{ m}) = 100 \text{ J}$. In choice (B), the work is equal to the change in gravitational potential energy: $W = mgh = (20 \text{ kg})(10 \text{ m/s}^2)(2 \text{ m}) = 400 \text{ J}$. In choice (C), there is no work done (though this is not easy to do!), since the person has caused no change in energy of the box. In choice (D), there is no work done against friction and no change in gravitational potential energy, so the work is equal to the change in the kinetic energy of the box: $W = \frac{1}{2}mv^2 = \frac{1}{2}(20 \text{ kg})(5 \text{ m/s})^2 = 250 \text{ J}$.

214. (D) The change in gravitational potential energy is equal to the gain in kinetic energy of the ball as the ball hits the floor. The floor does work on the ball in bringing it to a stop, so the ball does an equal amount of work on the floor (since the forces are equal and opposite).

$$mgh = \tfrac{1}{2}mv^2 = F_{\text{average}}d$$

$$(5 \text{ kg})(9.8 \text{ m/s}^2)(1 \text{ m}) = F(0.01 \text{ m})$$

$$F = 5{,}000 \text{ N}$$

215. (D) Power is the rate at which work is done or the rate at which energy is produced. In this case, the energy produced is the kinetic energy of the car after 20 s.

$$P = \frac{W}{t} = \frac{\Delta K}{\Delta t} = \frac{\tfrac{1}{2}mv^2}{t} = \frac{\tfrac{1}{2}(2000 \text{ kg})(40 \text{ m/s})^2}{20 \text{ s}} = 80{,}000 \text{ W, or } 80 \text{ kW}$$

The prefix *kilo-* means "1,000," so the answer is 80 kilowatts, sometimes abbreviated kW.

Another approach to this problem is to use the equation $P = Fv$, where F is average force and v is change in velocity, with force and velocity in the same direction. First, the acceleration is calculated ($a = \Delta v/\Delta t$), and then the force is calculated ($F = ma$). Finally, the force and the average velocity are applied to the power equation.

$$(1) \quad a = \frac{\Delta v}{\Delta t} = \frac{v_f - v_o}{t} = \frac{40 \text{ m/s} - 0}{20 \text{ s}} = 2 \text{ m/s}^2$$

$$(2) \quad F = ma = (2{,}000 \text{ kg})(2 \text{ m/s}^2) = 4{,}000 \text{ N}$$

$$(3) \quad P = Fv_{\text{average}} = (4{,}000 \text{ N})(20 \text{ m/s}) = 80{,}000 \text{ W}$$

216. (D) Power is the rate of energy use, or $P = E/t$. Therefore, the energy used is equal to power (in watts) times time (in seconds). Since there are 3,600 seconds in an hour, $3{,}600 \text{ s} \times 40 \text{ W} = 144{,}000 \text{ J}$.

217. (B) In choice (A), the speed doesn't change, so no work is done to increase kinetic or potential energy. However, there is work done against friction (the friction force (μmg) times the distance moved: $W = \mu mgd = (0.05)(20 \text{ kg})(10 \text{ N})(10 \text{ m/s}^2) = 100 \text{ J}$). The power generated is W/t, or 5 W. In choice (B), the work is equal to the change in gravitational potential energy: $W = mgh = (20 \text{ kg})(10 \text{ m/s}^2)(2 \text{ m}) = 400 \text{ J}$. The power generated is W/t, or 200 W. In choice (C), there is no work done (though this is not easy to do!), since the person has caused no change in energy of the box. In choice (D), there is no work done against friction and no change in gravitational potential energy, so the work is equal to the change in the kinetic energy of the box: $W = \tfrac{1}{2}mv^2 = \tfrac{1}{2}(20 \text{ kg})(5 \text{ m/s})^2 = 250 \text{ J}$. The power generated is W/t, or 25 W.

218. (A) There are two approaches to this problem.

(1) The change in kinetic energy of the object is calculated, then applied to the equation $P = \Delta K/t$, where ΔK is change in energy and t is time.

$$\Delta K = \tfrac{1}{2}m(v_f^2 - v_o^2) = \tfrac{1}{2}(2)(3^2 - 2^2) = 5 \text{ J}$$

$$P = \frac{\Delta K}{t} = \frac{5 \text{ J}}{10 \text{ s}} = 0.5 \text{ W}$$

(2) The equation $P = Fv$ is used, where F is average force and v is average velocity. If the acceleration is constant, it can be assumed that the force is constant and the average velocity is one half the sum of the initial and final velocities.

$$P = Fv = (0.2 \text{ N})\left(\frac{3 \text{ m/s} + 2 \text{ m/s}}{2}\right) = 0.5 \text{ W}$$

The equation $F = ma$ can also be used to calculate the acceleration. Once the acceleration is known, the distance it takes the force to accelerate the object the given amount is determined. The work done is calculated, and power is calculated as work divided by time.

219. (B) To keep the object moving at constant speed, enough power must be applied to the object so that the force moving the object forward is equal to the friction force of the surface on the object. The simplest approach is to calculate the friction force, then use the equation $P = Fv$.

$$F_f = \mu N = \mu mg = (0.2)(10 \text{ kg})(9.8 \text{ m/s}^2) = 20 \text{ N}$$
$$P = Fv = (20 \text{ N})(4.0 \text{ m/s}) = 80 \text{ W}$$

220. (B) Power is equal to energy divided by time, so the slope of the graph line is the average power.

$$\text{Slope} = \frac{\Delta y}{\Delta x} = \frac{100 \text{ J}}{10 \text{ s}} = 10 \text{ W}$$

Chapter 7: Thermodynamics

Note: The convention used throughout this book is that work done *on* a system is positive and work done *by* a system is negative. In this chapter, the first law of thermodynamics is expressed as $\Delta U = Q + W$, where U is internal energy, Q is energy transferred into (+) or out of (−) a system, and W is work—positive if performed *on* the system (a decrease in gas volume) and negative if performed *by* the system (an increase in gas volume).

221. (A) According to the first law of thermodynamics, two systems at different temperatures that come into contact will transfer energy until the system is at thermal equilibrium, at which point all parts of the system will be at the same temperature. There are more molecules in the larger cube, so the same energy absorbed by the larger cube produces a smaller change in average kinetic energy of molecules and thus a smaller temperature change.

222. (C) Thermal energy will be transferred from the higher-temperature block to the lower-temperature block until thermal equilibrium is reached, at which point both blocks will have the same temperature. Regardless of the material of which the blocks are composed, if they are at the same temperature, the average translational kinetic energy of molecules in both blocks will be the same.

223. (D) The term *isothermal* means that the temperature remains constant. Using the ideal gas equation $PV = nRT$, doubling the pressure while keeping the temperature constant has only one other possibility—reducing the volume to one half, which is not a choice.

224. (A) Using the ideal gas law, $PV = nRT$, the number of moles of gas in the container (n), the volume of the container (V), and the gas constant (R) do not change. Therefore, as the temperature (T) increases on one side of the equation, the pressure (P) increases on the other side of the equation; that is, as the temperature increases, with no change in volume, the average kinetic energy of the molecules increases. The molecules, on average, are moving faster and thus collide with the walls of the container with greater force and with a greater change in momentum.

$$F = \frac{m(v_f - v_o)}{t}$$

If the molecules collide with the walls of the container with greater force, the pressure increases.

$$\frac{F}{A} = P$$

225. (C) The first law of thermodynamics is $\Delta U = Q + W$, where U is the internal energy of the system, Q is heat added to or removed from the system, and positive W is work done *on* the system. If the process is adiabatic, by definition, Q is equal to zero and $\Delta U = W$. Internal energy, U, is proportional to the temperature of the system, so an increase in temperature, which is indicative of an increase in the average translational kinetic energy of molecules, must be due to work done on the system.

226. (A) Actual efficiency is equal to work output divided by heat input. If the engine takes in 475 J but rejects 315 J, the difference (160 J) must have been used to do work. Therefore, the actual efficiency is 160/475, or about one third, which is closest to 33.7% in choice (A).

Carnot efficiency is the difference between hot and cold temperatures divided by the hot temperature: $(750 - 250)/750 = 500/750 = 2/3$, or 66.7%.

227. (B) Using conservation of energy (the first law of thermodynamics), an increase in the internal energy of a system (ΔU) is equal to thermal energy added and/or work done on the system. The term *isothermal* means "no temperature change." Since internal energy is proportional to temperature, there is no change in internal energy during an isothermal process. Therefore, an amount of thermal energy must be added that is equal to the work done *by* the gas.

$$\Delta U = Q + W$$

Since $\Delta U = 0$, $Q = -W$.

228. (B) The molecules use the energy absorbed during the heating process to increase their kinetic energy. They have greater average speed, so collisions with the walls of the container are more frequent and exert more force on impact. However, since the container does not change in volume, the molecules do no work. Internal energy is directly proportional to change in temperature: $\Delta U = \frac{3}{2}nR\Delta T$. Therefore, choice (B) is correct. Choice (D) cannot be correct, because the root mean square speed of molecules increases with the square root of temperature; kinetic energy is directly proportional to temperature.

229. (A) The term *isothermal* means that there is no change in temperature during the process. The ideal gas equation is used: $PV = nRT$. Assuming that no molecules of the gas enter or leave the container (that is, the value of n, the number of moles of gas, does not change), it is concluded that P and V must be inversely proportional, since the value of nRT is constant. As P doubles, V is halved.

230. (C) Due to conservation of energy, described by the first law of thermodynamics, any change in internal energy is due to energy (Q) added or removed and/or work (W) done on or by the gas.

$$\Delta U = Q + W$$

Using the equation in this way, work done on the system is considered to be positive—and increases the internal energy of the gas. The net change in internal energy is the sum of the changes during the set of processes. Therefore, 80 J of work done on the gas increases the internal energy by the same amount. When the gas gives off 25 J of energy, that amount is subtracted from the internal energy. Then, when the gas does work on its surroundings, it uses some of its internal energy (40 J). The net change in internal energy is $\Delta U = +80$ J $- 25$ J $- 40$ J $= +15$ J.

231. (C) The internal energy of an ideal gas is proportional to the temperature and average kinetic energy of gas molecules. The first law of thermodynamics is the conservation of energy statement: $\Delta U = Q + W$, where U is internal energy, Q is heat, and W is work. An increase in internal energy would definitely be the result if heat is added to the system and work is done on the system, since each would increase internal energy. Choice (A) is not correct, because *isobaric* means that pressure remains constant, which could be true if work is done ($W = P\Delta V$); however, if during the process more heat is removed than work is done on the system, internal energy would decrease. Choice (B) is not correct, because no work is done if there is no change in volume (*isovolumetric* means that there is no change in volume). Choice (D) is not correct, because an isothermal process, by definition, means that there is no change in temperature and thus ΔV is zero.

232. (B) The change in entropy for each chamber can be estimated as heat transfer divided by average absolute temperature over which the transfer takes place: $\Delta S = Q/T_{average}$. Since the reservoirs are large, the transfer of only 500 J of energy in or out does not appreciably change the temperature of either chamber. Thus, the value of $T_{average}$ can be assumed not to change during the transfer. The hotter chamber has a higher average temperature; when T is larger, ΔS is smaller (since Q is the same for both chambers). The hotter chamber, then, undergoes a smaller change in entropy, and the cooler chamber undergoes a larger change in entropy. Additionally, the net change in entropy of the universe is the sum of the two entropy changes. The cooler chamber has heat transferred in, so the value of Q is positive and the value for entropy change is positive. The entropy change for the hotter chamber is negative, since heat is transferred out. The sum of the entropy changes is positive, so the net entropy change for this process is positive. The entropy of the universe increases as a result.

233. (D) Without using calculus, the change in entropy of a system is estimated as heat transferred in or out of a system divided by the average Kelvin temperature during the process.

$$\Delta S = \frac{Q}{T_{average(K)}}$$

The change in entropy for Chamber X is $-Q$ divided by T_1. Q is negative, since the heat is transferred out—from higher temperature to lower temperature. The change in entropy for Chamber Y is $+Q/T_2$. The value of Q is the same for both chambers. However, since T_1 is higher than T_2, the change is entropy in the first case is lower. The negative sign can be ignored, because the focus is on magnitudes. Thus, Chamber X loses the same amount of heat as Chamber Y gains, but the change in entropy for Chamber X is less than the change in entropy for Chamber Y.

234. (A) The boiling water inside the beaker will stay hot longest when the product of conductivity (k) and thermal gradient (ΔT) is least for the insulating liquid so that transfer of energy by conduction is minimized. These two variables are found in the following equation.

$$\frac{Q}{t} = \frac{kA\Delta T}{L}$$

Considering that all the other parameters are about the same, the liquid for the bath is selected such that the product of k and ΔT (the difference between the liquid temperature and the temperature of boiling water at 100°C) is smallest. In choice (A), the product is 0.145 W/m·C° × 10°C, or 1.45 W/m. In choice (B), the product is 0.202 W/m·C° × 20°C, or 4.03 W/m. In choice (C), the product is 0.609 W/m·C° × 10°C, or 6.09 W/m. In choice (D), the product is 0.609 W/m·C° × 20°C, or 12.18 W/m. Of these, the smallest heat transfer rate (in joules per second per meter of liquid surrounding the beaker) is to the oil in choice (A).

235. (B) Convection takes place in fluids, that is, in liquids and gases. As a fluid is heated, it expands, becomes less dense, and then rises—allowing cooler, more dense fluid to sink under the influence of gravity (since it is more dense).

236. (B) The rate at which heat is transferred from a higher temperature reservoir to a lower temperature reservoir is calculated as follows.

$$\frac{Q}{t} = \frac{kA\Delta T}{L}$$

where Q/t is the rate of heat transfer, k is the conductivity of the material used (in this case, silver, which has high conductivity), A is the cross-sectional area through which energy is transferred by conduction, ΔT is the temperature difference between the hot and cold regions, and L is the length through which the energy is transferred. Doubling A and halving L would increase the rate of transfer most.

237. (C) The rate at which heat is transferred by conduction through a steel rod is directly proportional to the thermal conductivity, cross-sectional area, and difference in temperature between the two chambers, and inversely proportional to the length of the rod. Choice (A) is not correct, because specific heat is not the correct quantity to use here. Choice (B) is not correct, because making these changes in temperature in the two chambers would decrease the temperature difference between the chambers, which would decrease the rate of heat flow through the rod. Choice (D), in which the cross-sectional area is decreased, would decrease the rate of heat transfer by conduction.

238. (B) Infrared radiation is electromagnetic radiation. When you put your hand near a warm stove, you are sensing infrared radiation, which is not in the visible range.

239. (D) It is important to realize that the kinetic energy is transferred by conduction, but that individual molecules do not actually travel from one end of the spoon to the other.

240. (D) The rate of energy transfer through the door by conduction is calculated, using Q for heat, t for time, k for thermal conductivity, A for the area of the door, T for temperature, and d for the thickness of the door.

$$\frac{\Delta Q}{\Delta t} = \frac{kA\Delta T}{d} = \frac{(0.1 \text{ W/m·C°})(2.0 \text{ m})(1.0 \text{ m})(50 \text{ C°})}{0.02 \text{ m}} = 500 \text{ W}$$

This result, 500 watts, is the same as 500 J/s. As the formula shows, the rate at which heat is transferred through the door by conduction increases with the area of the door and the temperature difference between inside and outside. Heat transfer decreases as the thickness of the door increases.

241. (C) Electrical resistance increases with temperature for most materials. The speed of sound in air increases with temperature. As temperature increases, the volume of a gas is expected to increase; however, if the number of molecules is constant and mass is constant, density (mass divided by volume) would be expected to decrease with temperature. Using the equation $PV = nRT$, if volume is kept constant, pressure would be expected to increase with temperature. Most solid objects increase in length with temperature.

242. (B) Since the ball and the ring are made of the same material, they have the same coefficient of expansion and thus expand at the same rate. The diameter of the ball and the diameter of the ring increase the same amount, so the ball will fit through the ring as the two are heated together.

243. (C) To determine the change in length of an object when it expands during heating, the following formula is used.

$$\Delta L = \alpha L_o \Delta T = (12 \times 10^{-6}/\text{C}°)(1 \text{ cm})(30°\text{C}) = 0.00036 \text{ cm}$$

$$\% \text{ change} = \frac{\Delta L}{L_o} = \frac{0.00036}{1} \times 100\% = 0.036\%$$

244. (B) The key to solving this problem is the approximation that the coefficient of area expansion for a material is twice the coefficient of linear expansion. The original area of the plate is equal to $(0.1 \text{ m})^2$, or 0.01 m^2. This area is applied to the formula for expansion.

$$A_f = A_o + \Delta A = A_o + 2\alpha A_o \Delta T$$
$$A_f = (100 \text{ cm}^2) + (20 \times 10^{-6}/\text{C}°)(100 \text{ cm}^2)(10°\text{C}) = 100.02 \text{ cm}^2$$

245. (A) Work done on an ideal gas causes a compression, or decrease, in the volume of the gas ($W = -P\Delta V$). There is no change in volume in steps II and IV, so no work is done on or by the gas molecules in either of those steps. In step III, the gas expands, so work is done by the gas in expanding itself. Only step I shows a decrease in volume, which means work was done by an external force in compressing the system of gas molecules.

246. (C) Conservation of energy is described by the first law of thermodynamics: $\Delta U = Q + W$. One complete cycle, starting at state A and returning the gas to state A, brings the gas back to its original conditions of pressure and volume. The ideal gas law, $PV = nRT$, indicates that if P and V are unchanged after the cycle, then T has also returned to its original value. If temperature doesn't change, then internal energy doesn't change ($\Delta U = \frac{3}{2}nR\Delta T$). Returning to the first law equation, if ΔU is zero, then $Q = -W$ for a complete cycle. The work for a complete cycle is the area confined by the closed curve. Since this is a triangle, $W = \text{area} = \frac{1}{2}bh = \frac{1}{2}(3 \text{ m}^3)(3,000 \text{ Pa}) = 4,500 \text{ J}$.

In this cycle, where work is the area between the line and the volume axis, the work during step AB is an expansion, which is larger than the work during step BC. Step AB is work done *by* the gas, and step BC is work done *on* the gas. No work is done on or by the gas in step CA, since there is no change in volume ($W = P\Delta V$). Therefore, the net work done by the gas requires energy, which means that energy must be added for this cycle. This work is equal in magnitude to the heat exchange, which is 4,500 J.

247. (C) Internal energy change for the complete cycle is zero, since the system is back to its original state conditions of P, V, and T. Since $\Delta U = Q + W$, the work for the complete cycle is equal to Q for the cycle. By the convention used here, expansion of the gas or work done by the gas on its surroundings is negative. There is more work done by the gas in expanding in step BC than the positive work done in compressing the gas in step CA, so the net work in this complete cycle is negative. Using the equation above, $W = -Q$, so if the work for the cycle is negative, then Q for the entire cycle is positive (that is, energy has been added). Now, add the heat changes given in the problem.

$$Q = 78 - 50 - 20 = 8 \text{ J}$$
$$W = -Q = -8 \text{ J}$$

The net work for the cycle is the work done during step BC (negative) plus the work done during step CA, which is the area under the line BC.

$W_{net} = -8 \text{ kJ} = W_{BC} - W_{CA}$

$W_{CA} = (4 \text{ m}^3)(1 \text{ kPa}) = 4 \text{ kJ}$

$W_{BC} = -12 \text{ kJ}$

248. (B) On a Pressure as a Function of Volume (PV) diagram, the net work done on or by the gas can be estimated by the area enclosed by the cycle. In this case, the work during step AB is done by the gas, since the gas expands in volume during this step. In step BC, no work is done on or by the gas, since there is no change in volume ($W = -P\Delta V$). During step CA, the gas is compressed by an external force, so volume decreases and work is done on the gas. It is in step CA that the most work is done on the gas. In each step, the area between the curve and the volume axis represents the amount of work done. Summing these areas and giving work done by the gas the opposite sign of the work done on the gas, the area enclosed represents the net work done. The area is approximately the area of a triangle: $\frac{1}{2}(1.5 \text{ m}^3)(8{,}000 \text{ Pa}) = 6{,}000 \text{ J}$.

249. (A) Step CA is isobaric, since the pressure is constant along that line. Step BC is isovolumetric, since the volume is constant during that step. Both isothermal processes and adiabatic processes are curves on a PV diagram, so it remains to determine which of these is represented by step AB. An isothermal process is one during which the temperature does not change. Using the ideal gas equation $PV = nRT$, the values for n, R, and T would all be constant for an isothermal process; therefore, the product of P and V would also have to be constant. Using the values of P and V on the diagram, it is apparent that the product of the two is 5,000 all along the line, so the line is isothermal.

250. (D) The energy conservation law is applied to each step: $\Delta U = Q + W$, where U is internal energy, Q is energy transferred in or out of the gas, and W is work done on the gas. For a step to be adiabatic, Q must be zero. Step AB is isovolumetric, and since $W = P\Delta V$, work must be zero. The temperature must increase in step AB (since P increases and $V = 0$), so U increases. Therefore, Q cannot be zero in step AB.

In step BC, the temperature is constant. Since internal energy is proportional to temperature ($U = \frac{3}{2}nRT$), ΔU must be zero. Since there is a volume change and work is done by the gas in expansion during this step, W is not zero and Q cannot be zero.

In step CA, the volume decreases, so work is done on the system in compressing the gas. By the definition used above, this is positive work. However, the temperature must decrease, since V does not change and P decreases ($PV = nRT$); therefore, U decreases. In the equation above, Q must have a negative value in this step for conservation of energy (ΔU is negative and W is positive).

None of these processes can be adiabatic. An adiabatic process on a PV diagram is a curve much like the isothermal line for step BC, except that an adiabatic curve dips much lower as the temperature of the gas drops quickly during expansion.

Chapter 8: Periodic Motion, Mechanical Waves, and Sound

251. (B) The acceleration of the pendulum bob is zero when the net force on it is zero ($\Sigma F = ma$). The net force is zero when the pendulum bob is at the bottom of its swing, that is, when its displacement is zero.

252. (A) The distance the spring is displaced defines the spring's amplitude, which does not affect the period or frequency. Period depends only on the mass and spring constant.

$$T = 2\pi\sqrt{\frac{m}{k}}$$

253. (C) The mass attached to a pendulum does not affect the period. Doubling the length will increase the period by a factor of $\sqrt{2}$, according the following equation.

$$T = 2\pi\sqrt{\frac{L}{g}}$$

254. (D) At the lowest point of its vertical oscillation, the object is at its amplitude, or at a maximum displacement from equilibrium. (The other point during its oscillation when it is at its maximum displacement is at the top.) Also at its lowest point, the object is causing the greatest extension of the spring, so the force exerted by the spring on the object is maximum, and thus acceleration is a maximum ($F = ma$). However, at its lowest point, the velocity of the object is zero, since the energy of the spring-mass system is all in the form of potential energy, and kinetic energy is zero. Thus, choice (D) is the correct combination. At the equilibrium position, the velocity is maximum, acceleration is zero, and displacement is zero.

255. (D) The period and frequency of oscillation of a simple harmonic oscillator, such as a mass oscillating on a spring, do not depend on the amplitude of the oscillation. As a spring oscillates, friction will gradually do negative work on the spring, reducing the total amount of mechanical energy in the spring-mass system. However, even though the energy decreases—and the amplitude decreases with it—the frequency and period of the oscillations remain the same until the oscillator comes to a complete stop.

256. (B) The equation describing a simple harmonic oscillator is of the form $x(t) = A \cos (2\pi ft)$, where A is the amplitude and f is the frequency of the oscillation. The cosine function simply means that the oscillator is at A (its amplitude) when $t = 0$. If the spring has a period of 0.5 s, the frequency of its oscillation is 2 Hz ($T = 1/f$). With an amplitude of 4 m, only choices (B) and (D) could be correct. If the frequency is 2 s, then $2\pi f$ equals 4π, so only choice (B) could be correct.

257. (A) The general form is $x(t) = A \cos (2\pi ft)$ or $x(t) = A \sin (2\pi ft)$, depending on the position of the oscillator when $t = 0$. In this problem, the amplitude, A, is equal to 2.5 m, so only choices (A) and (B) are possible. Since $2\pi f$ is equal to 4 and $f = 1/T$, $2\pi/T = 4$. Then $T = 2\pi/4$, or $\pi/2$.

258. (A) As the mass on the spring oscillates, its velocity is zero at the amplitude of the oscillation, or where the mass "turns" to change direction, much like a ball thrown into the air turns to come back down. The velocity is zero, then, at the times 2 s, 6 s, 10 s, 14 s, 18 s, and 22 s on the graph.

Another approach to this problem is to consider that the velocity is zero when the kinetic energy is zero; at the amplitude of its oscillation, the potential energy of the oscillator is maximum, so kinetic energy is zero.

259. (C) According to Hooke's law, $F = -kx$, with the negative sign indicating that the spring force, F, and the displacement, x, are in opposite directions. According to Newton's second law of motion, $F = ma$, force and acceleration are in the same direction. Combining these two laws, the displacement of the mass and acceleration of the mass must be in opposite directions. However, the displacement is zero at 0 and 4 seconds, so it has no direction. Answer choice (C) is the only possibility.

260. (A) A *transverse* wave is one in which the oscillations of particles of a medium are perpendicular to the direction of propagation of the medium. A *longitudinal* wave is one in which the oscillations of a medium are along the same direction as the direction of propagation of the wave; sound is an example of a longitudinal wave. A *compressional* wave describes the compression of a longitudinal wave. The term *spherical* describes the shape of a wave front, not a type of wave.

261. (A) The waves travel from A to B, transferring energy to the person's ear, which makes the eardrum oscillate so that the person can hear the sound. However, the air molecules oscillate within a confined space, so the molecules transfer energy from one to another—much like a lineup of dominoes—but the molecules don't travel beyond the amplitudes of their oscillations in place. Choice (C) describes a transverse oscillation, which is not the means by which sound travels. Choice (D) is not correct; the frequency remains the same, which defines the pitch of the sound. The amplitude may decrease with distance, however, causing the sound to be less loud as it travels farther.

262. (C) Blowing through an instrument increases the temperature of the air inside the instrument, which increases the speed of sound in the air inside the instrument. Assuming very little change in the dimensions of the instrument itself during the warming-up process, the wavelengths produced by specific notes would not change. Therefore, using the equation $v = f\lambda$, an increase in the speed of sound would produce a corresponding increase in the frequency. Humans perceive an increase in frequency as higher "pitch."

263. (C) The two waves have the same amplitude, about 2 units. Wave A has a period of about 3 s—the time for one complete oscillation. Frequency is the inverse of period, so wave A has a frequency of ⅓ Hz. Wave B has a period of about 2 s and a frequency of ½ Hz, so the frequency of wave B is higher than that of wave A. At about 3.8 s, the waves meet at crest and trough, where they would destructively interfere. At 4.2 seconds, the wave amplitudes are both zero, so they don't interfere. At 8.0 s, the waves are both in the same position, or in phase, so they constructively interfere.

264. (A) A maximum occurs at point B, because the distance from each opening to point B is the same. Thus, the waves are still in phase with each other—and constructively interfere—at point B. For a maximum, or constructive interference of the waves, to occur at point A, the extra distance the waves from one slit have to travel to point A compared to the distance the waves travel from the other slit must be one wavelength; this is called the path length difference. For constructive interference, the path length difference must be a whole number of wavelengths so that the waves are in phase when they meet at that point.

265. (C) Waves are in the same phase when they are in the same position, that is, at the same amplitude and traveling in the same direction. The two oscillations start in the same position at $t = 0$, with an amplitude of 0 and moving toward the positive direction. In choice (A), wave A is at 0 and moving toward the positive direction, while wave B is at 0 and moving toward the negative direction. In choice (B), wave A is at an amplitude of 2 and wave B is at an amplitude of -2. In choice (C), waves A and B are both at an amplitude of about -2 and moving toward the same direction, so they are in phase. In choice (D), wave A is near a maximum positive amplitude and wave B is near zero.

266. (A) Moving the speaker twice as far away reduces the intensity to one fourth, since intensity of sound varies as the inverse square of distance. However, doubling the intensity at the source brings the intensity from one fourth to one half of the original.

267. (C) The value for intensity is substituted into the equation and easily calculated, since it is known that $\log 100 = 2$.

$$\beta = 10 \log \frac{I}{I_o} = 10 \log \frac{1 \times 10^{-10}}{1 \times 10^{-12}} = 10 \log 100 = 10(2) = 20 \text{ dB}$$

268. (C) Intensity is multiplied by 10 when the decibel level increases by 10. The proof is shown below, where the intensity, I, for 50 decibels is 1×10^{-7} W/m² and the intensity for 60 decibels is 1×10^{-6} W/m².

$$\beta = 10 \log \frac{I}{I_o} = 60 = 10(6) = 10 \log 10^6 = 10 \log \frac{1 \times 10^{-6}}{1 \times 10^{-12}}$$

$$\beta = 10 \log \frac{I}{I_o} = 50 = 10(5) = 10 \log 10^5 = 10 \log \frac{1 \times 10^{-7}}{1 \times 10^{-12}}$$

269. (B) When the waves are added, or superimposed, their amplitudes at that point in time are summed. At $t = 0$, the sum of the two amplitudes is $0 + 2$, or 2 m. At $t = 7$, the sum of the two amplitudes is approximately $1.5 + 1.5$, or 3 m. At $t = 9$, the sum of the two amplitudes is $0 + -2$, or -2 m. At $t = 12$, the sum of the two amplitudes is approximately $1.5 + -1$, or 0.5 m.

270. (D) The amplitude will add to zero when the centers of peaks of the waves are in the same position. Each wave is 1 m wide, so they completely cancel when the centers are in the same position. At the point shown in the graph, the centers are at $x = 2.5$ and $x = 9.5$, so the centers are 7 m apart. Each wave covers half this distance, so it is necessary to determine the time for the pulses to travel 3.5 m: $t = d/v = 3.5$ m/5 m/s = about 0.7 s.

271. (B) The peaks of the two pulses completely overlap to produce a wave of the greatest amplitude when each pulse has moved 0.75 m. This puts the peak of pulse A between $x = 1.25$ and $x = 1.5$ and the peak of pulse B between $x = 1.25$ and $x = 1.5$. The waves would overlap as they pass that position, producing a pulse of double amplitude. Since the pulses are moving at the same speed, they will reach that position at $t = d/v = 0.75$ m/ 2 m/s $= 0.375$ s.

272. (C) The sound is a maximum at the original position, because the waves have traveled the same distance from each speaker, are in phase, and constructively interfere. At the second position, the sound waves from the two speakers destructively interfere, so the waves are ½ wavelength, or 180°, out of phase. Therefore, the wavelength must be some multiple of 1 m: 1 m, 2 m, 3 m, and so on.

273. (D) The standing wave produced in the open tube has antinodes at both ends and a node in the middle, so the fundamental standing wave in the tube is ½ wavelength. The fundamental wavelength is $2L$. The equation $v = f\lambda$ is used to determine the frequency: $f = v/\lambda$. Substitution yields $f = v/2L$.

274. (D) The standing wave produced in the closed tube has a node at the closed end and an antinode at the open end, so the fundamental standing wave in the tube is ¼ wavelength. The fundamental wavelength is four times the length of the tube. The equation $v = f\lambda$ is used to determine the frequency: $f = v/\lambda$. Substitution yields $f = v/4L$. Using the same process, the wavelength for the open tube is two times the length of the tube, so the frequency equals $v/2L$. The frequency for the closed tube is one half the frequency for the open tube. Of two frequencies, the one that is lower in number is said to have a lower pitch. In fact, when the frequency is half of the other, it is an octave lower.

275. (D) The harmonics for the tube closed at one end, where the standing wave has a node at one end and an antinode at the other end, are calculated as follows.

$$\lambda_n = \frac{4L}{n}$$

where $n = 1, 3, 5$, etc.

The harmonics in a tube open at both ends are calculated in the same way as the harmonics for a string attached at both ends.

$$\lambda_n = \frac{2L}{n}$$

The wavelength for the first harmonic for the closed tube is twice as long as the wavelength for the open tube. Therefore, a closed tube that is half as long as an open tube would produce notes of the same wavelength and frequency.

276. (D) The general formula for wavelength related to the length on which the standing wave is confined (for a string attached at both ends or a tube open at both ends) is $\lambda = 2L/n$, where n is the number of the harmonic. The first and second overtones are the second and third harmonics (since the fundamental is the first harmonic). Because $v = f\lambda$, the information given is used to determine v for the string: $v = f\lambda = 2fL/n = 2(200)(.4)/1 = 160$ m/s. This value of v can be used to determine the other two harmonics. The second harmonic (the first overtone) is determined from the equation $160 = 2f(.4)/2$; $f = 400$ Hz. The third harmonic (the second overtone) is determined from the equation $160 = 2f(.4)/3$; $f = 600$ Hz. The harmonics for a string fixed at both ends or a tube open at both ends are multiples of the fundamental frequency.

277. (D) The general formula for wavelength related to the length on which the standing wave is confined for a tube closed at one end is $\lambda = 4L/n$, where n must be an odd number. For the fundamental, $n = 1$, and $n = 3$ and $n = 5$ for the next two overtones. Because $v = f\lambda$, the information given is used to determine v for the air in the tube: $v = f\lambda = 4fL/n = 4(100)(.8)/1 = 320$ m/s. This value of v can be used to determine the other two overtones. The first overtone (the third harmonic) is determined from the equation $320 = 4f(.8)/3$; $f = 300$ Hz. (Note: A calculator is not required for this computation—the fractions are simply compared: n is 3 times as much, so f is 3 times as much.) The second overtone (the fifth harmonic) is determined from the equation $320 = 4f(.8)/5$; $f = 500$ Hz. The harmonics for a tube open at only one end are odd-number multiples of the fundamental frequency. The harmonics for this closed tube are 100 Hz (fundamental), 300 Hz, and 500 Hz.

278. (C) An open tube has harmonic frequencies that are multiples of the fundamental frequency, so the next higher frequency at which the open tube will resonate is the second harmonic, which has twice the frequency of the fundamental (or first harmonic). A closed tube has harmonics that follow the odd numbers, so the frequency of the next harmonic is three times the frequency of the fundamental (or first harmonic). (The harmonic after that has five times the fundamental frequency, and so on.) Interestingly, the harmonics for a string attached at both ends are identical to the harmonics for a tube that is open at both ends.

279. (C) Assuming that the speed of sound is the same for the tube at both lengths, for a tube closed at one end, the fundamental wavelength is $4L$. Since $v = f\lambda$, $f = v/\lambda = v/4L$. After the tube is cut in half, the length is $L/2$, so $f = v/4(L/2) = v/2L$. The frequency of the shorter tube is twice the frequency of the original tube.

280. (C) To increase the number of loops in the standing wave, the wavelength of the standing wave needs to be shortened. Because $v = f\lambda$, this can be accomplished by any action that increases the frequency while maintaining the wave speed or decreasing the wave speed while maintaining the frequency. In the correct choice (C), loosening the string to decrease the tension would decrease the speed of waves on the string. (The speed of a wave on a string is directly proportional to the tension in the string and inversely proportional to the linear density of the string.) When wave speed is decreased and all other factors are the same, the wavelength will decrease, so more loops can be produced on the string. Choice (A) is not correct, because decreasing frequency would increase the wavelength if wave speed were kept constant. Choice (B) is not correct, because a thinner string would have a lower linear density, which would increase the speed of waves on the string, which would increase the wavelength if the frequency were maintained. Choice (D) is not correct, because moving the supports apart will not change the number of loops.

281. (A) As the two frequencies superimpose, there are positions where the waves meet in the same phase, reinforcing and producing constructive interference—six times per second. In between, the waves from the two tuning forks are not in phase and destructively interfere, producing sound that is partially or completely "canceled." This pattern of higher amplitude and constructive interference six times per second is called the beat frequency.

282. (C) The addition of clay to two of the tuning forks increased the period and decreased the frequency—much like lengthening a pendulum. The difference in frequency of one of the modified tuning forks and the original will be the number of beats heard per second. Five beats per second between X and modified Y indicate that Y has a frequency 5 Hz less than X. A beat frequency of three beats per second heard between Y and Z means that Y and Z are 3 Hz different in frequency. Without knowing how much clay was added to Y and Z, however, it cannot be determined which has the higher frequency. Z could be lower in frequency than Y and, therefore, a total of 8 Hz lower than X, or Z could be higher in frequency than Y and, therefore, a total of 2 Hz lower than X.

283. (A) As the truck approaches, the perceived frequency of the sound produced by the trombone will increase, so the frequency of the A note played by the trombone in the truck will be higher than the A note being played by the saxophone on the street corner. The beat frequency is the difference in frequency of the two notes being superimposed, so the note played by the trombone in the truck must be 4 Hz higher, or 444 Hz. This is an example of the Doppler effect.

284. (C) An interference frequency of 4 beats per second means the two sounds differ in frequency by 4 Hz. Sanding one pipe to make it shorter decreases the wavelength of the standing wave produced by the pipe, and a decrease in wavelength means an increase in frequency. (This assumes that the speed of sound is the same in both pipes, and $v = f\lambda$.) Therefore, the shorter pipe would have a frequency of 260 + 4, or 264 Hz.

285. (A) When the instrument is tuned, the length of the air column inside the instrument is set, so that the fundamental wavelength for that note does not change until the instrument is tuned again. However, as the air in the clarinet becomes warmer, the velocity of sound increases, using the equation $v_{air} = 331$ m/s $+ 0.6\ T_C$. The equation $v = f\lambda$, where v is the speed of sound, f is the frequency of the note, and λ is the fundamental wavelength of the note, is applied. If wavelength is constant, then frequency must increase as the temperature and velocity increase. As a result, a wind instrument will tend to go up in frequency—or play the notes "sharp"—unless the instrument is warmed up well before playing.

286. (D) As sound travels from one medium to another in which the speed of sound is different, the waves may change direction, a phenomenon called *refraction*. This happens at night, for example, near the surface of Earth over bodies of water. The air is cooler over the water, and sound travels more slowly in cooler air. Sounds traveling away from a source bend downward toward the cooler air near the surface, so the sounds may seem amplified.

287. (B) Attenuation of sound in fluids is directly proportional to the frequency of the sound and the viscosity of the medium. (In fact, it is usually proportional to the square of the sound frequency.) Attenuation varies inversely with the density of the medium and the speed of sound in that medium.

288. (D) The speed of sound in air increases with elasticity and decreases with density, according to the following equation.

$$v = \sqrt{\frac{B}{\rho}}$$

where B is the elastic modulus and ρ is density. Since increasing the temperature makes air more elastic and decreases its density, a temperature increase directly increases the speed of sound.

289. (B) The diffraction, or bending, of sound waves around the corner of a building allows you to hear sounds from objects that you cannot see. (Light also diffracts, but the much shorter wavelengths for light make this phenomenon of a much smaller magnitude.) Choice (A) is an example of the attenuation of sound as it is absorbed and scattered by the medium. Choice (C) is an example of the Doppler effect, or an increase in frequency when a sound source moves toward a stationary observer. Choice (D) is an example of the decrease of sound speed in colder air; this effect is much less noticeable on a warm day, when sound travels faster.

290. (B) The attenuation coefficient varies widely for different materials, so ultrasonic signals can be used to reveal structural information in many different contexts, from the human fetus to the chemical composition of solutions.

291. (C) The Doppler effect will be greatest when the relative velocity between the sound source and the observer is greatest. In choice (A), where the siren is moving closer, the perceived frequency is higher than the siren frequency. In choice (B), where the siren and observer are separating at the same speed as in choice (A), the perceived frequency is lower than the siren frequency. Generally speaking, however, the Doppler effect is greater when the source is moving relative to a stationary observer than when the observer is moving relative to a stationary source. In choice (C), the siren and observer are both approaching the intersection at a speed of 30 m/s; using a right-triangle relationship, these speeds are the legs of a triangle with a hypotenuse of approximately 42. Therefore, the observer and siren are approaching each other at a rate of 42 m/s, which produces the greatest effect. In choice (D), the observer is moving away from the intersection at 30 m/s and the siren is moving toward the intersection in the same direction at 30 m/s. In this case, they are not closing in or receding from each other, so the relative velocity is zero and there is no Doppler effect.

In another approach to calculating the situation in choice (C), the difference is the resultant of the siren vector (from the east) and the negative of the observer vector (toward the south), as shown.

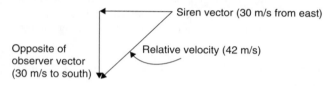

292. (C) You will hear a higher frequency from the siren when the two vehicles are moving toward each other with the highest relative speed. When the vehicles are moving away from each other, you will hear a lower frequency than the siren is emitting. In choice (C), the highest relative speed occurs, because you are moving toward the siren and the siren is moving toward you.

In choice (D), the two vehicles are moving in the same direction at the same speed, so there is no relative speed and you will hear the same frequency that the siren is emitting.

293. (D) Choice (A) is not possible, since the wavelength range for sound, even for very high frequencies, is many orders of magnitude too large to interact directly with molecules. Both choices (B) and (C) are viable.

294. (A) Ultrasonic has all the properties of sound, except that it is in the range of frequency higher than 20,000 Hz—beyond the range of human hearing. It should not be confused with supersonic, which means traveling faster than the speed of sound in a given medium.

Chapter 9: Fluids and Solids

295. (B) Density is equal to mass divided by volume. Since the piece of halite is submerged, the volume of oil displaced by it is the volume of the sample. The density of the oil is not a factor in this calculation.

$$\rho = \frac{m}{V} = \frac{220 \text{ g}}{100 \text{ cm}^3} = 2.2 \text{ g/cm}^3$$

296. (B) If the block of wood floats 60% below the surface of water, the block has a density 60% that of water (which is 1,000 kg/m³); thus, the block's density is 600 kg/m³. If the alcohol is 90% as dense as water, the alcohol's density is 900 kg/m³. Consequently, the block's density is 600/900 that of alcohol, so the block should float in the alcohol so that it is two thirds under the surface. This is logical, since the block will have to submerge slightly more in alcohol to displace enough alcohol to create a buoyant force equal to the block's weight.

297. (B) The weight of fluid displaced by an object partially or fully submerged in the fluid is equal to the buoyant force of the fluid on that object. When an object floats, the buoyant force is equal to the object's weight in air. If the object floats only 75% submerged, then the object must displace only three quarters of its volume in order to displace a volume of fluid that weighs the same as the object weighs in air. Density equals mass divided by volume: $\rho = m/V$.

To express this concept differently: a volume of fluid that is 75% of the volume of an object weighs the same as the entire object. Thus, the fluid must be four thirds the density of the object and the object's density is three quarters that of the fluid. As a general rule, for an object that floats in a fluid, the depth to which the object floats indicates the ratio of the density of the object to the density of the fluid.

298. (A) Liquid A has a specific gravity of 0.5, so it has a density that is half the density of water, or 500 kg/m³. If we know the density and volume of liquid A, we can determine its mass. (Note: 1 ml is about 1 cm³, which is 1×10^{-6} m³.)

$$\rho = \frac{m}{V}$$

$$m = \rho V = (500 \text{ kg/m}^3)(60 \times 10^{-6} \text{ m}^3) = 0.03 \text{ kg}$$

Next, the mass of liquid B is determined.

$$m = \rho V = (700 \text{ kg/m}^3)(40 \times 10^{-6} \text{ m}^3) = 0.028 \text{ kg}$$

Then, the total mass and total volume are used to determine the density of the solution.

$$\rho = \frac{m}{V} = \frac{0.058 \text{ kg}}{100 \text{ ml}} = \frac{0.058 \text{ kg}}{100 \times 10^{-6} \text{ m}^3} = 580 \text{ kg/m}^3$$

$$SG = \frac{\rho_{solution}}{\rho_{water}} = \frac{580 \text{ kg/m}^3}{1,000 \text{ kg/m}^3} = 0.58$$

299. (D) Choice (D) is a statement of Archimedes' principle, in the sense that the weight of fluid displaced by the ball is equal to the buoyant force of the fluid on the ball. If the ball floats, the forces on the ball are in equilibrium, so the gravitational force on the ball (its weight in air) is equal to the buoyant force of the fluid on the ball. Since the ball must have only half of its volume submerged in order to displace a weight of fluid equal to the ball's weight, the ball must be only half as dense as the fluid (density = mass/volume). The weight of the ball equals the weight of the fluid displaced; the volume of the fluid is half the volume of the ball and the density of the fluid is twice the density of the ball.

300. (B) If the block has a density very close to the density of water and is at room temperature, it would sink in hot water. Hot water is less dense than water at room temperature, so the block would be more dense than the water and therefore sink. As the block warms in the hot water, it also becomes less dense and closer to the density of the water, so it will rise and float. The warm block will float in the second container of water if the water in that container is quite cold. As the water approaches room temperature, the block cools and becomes more dense, so the block rises and floats. The block is evidently slightly less dense than water when both are at room temperature.

301. (D) There are three forces on the rock when it is under water: a spring force upward, a buoyant force upward, and the gravitational force downward. The buoyant force is equal to the weight of water displaced (10 ml, or 10 g, of water): $W = mg = (0.01 \text{ kg})(9.8 \text{ m/s}^2)$ $= 0.098$ N. The weight of the rock is equal to the spring force plus the buoyant force: $W = 0.80$ N $+ 0.098$ N $= 0.9$ N. The mass of the rock is its weight divided by g: $m = W/g = 0.9$ N$/9.8$ m/s$^2 = 0.09$ kg (90 grams).

Another approach to this problem is to consider that the apparent loss of weight of the rock when it is submerged is equal to the buoyant force on the rock. The buoyant force on a submerged object is equal to $\rho V g$, where ρ is the density of the water and V is the volume of water displaced. Therefore, the buoyant force is calculated as follows.

$$F = \rho V g = (1{,}000 \text{ kg/m}^3)(10 \times 10^{-6} \text{ m}^3)(9.8 \text{ m/s}^2) = 0.1 \text{ N}$$

The weight of the rock is the buoyant force plus the spring force, or 0.9 N. The mass of the rock is 0.9 N divided by g, which is 0.09 kg, or 90 g.

302. (C) The fact that the ball floats 60% below the surface in water means that it must sink only that far to displace enough water to weigh the same as the ball's weight. Therefore, the ball is 60% as dense as water, and its density is 600 kg/m^3. The ball sinks 70% below the surface in the second liquid, so the ball is 70% as dense as the second liquid. The density of the ball, then, is 0.7 times the density of the second liquid: $0.7\rho = 600$ kg/m^3. The density of the second liquid is about 860 kg/m^3.

303. (B) Since the bar is in equilibrium, the net force in the vertical direction is zero. The two tension forces, $2T$, are upward, and so is the buoyant force on the bar. The gravitational force, W, is the same whether the bar is in or out of water, so $2T + F = W$.

304. (B) If the ball floats, it is in equilibrium, with the buoyant force equal to the weight of the ball.

$$F_B = mg = (0.020 \text{ kg})(9.8 \text{ m/s}^2) = 0.196 \text{ N}$$

305. (A) The total fluid pressure in each side of the tube is the same at equilibrium. The total pressure of water plus oil plus atmospheric pressure on the left side must equal the total pressure of water plus atmospheric pressure on the right side. Since atmospheric pressure is essentially the same on both sides, only the pressure due to oil and water needs to be considered.

$$P_{oil} + P_{water \text{ (left)}} = P_{water \text{ (right)}}$$

$$\rho_{oil} h_{oil} + \rho_{water} h_{water \text{ (left)}} = \rho_{water} h_{water \text{ (right)}}$$

$\rho_{oil}(0.08 \text{ m}) + (1,000 \text{ kg/m}^3)(0.20 \text{ m}) = (1,000 \text{ kg/m}^3)(0.25 \text{ m})$

$\rho_{oil} = 600 \text{ kg/m}^3$

A quick method of working this problem is based on the recognition that 8 cm of oil must have the same fluid pressure as 5 cm of water. Therefore, the oil is ⅝ as dense as water. Since the density of water is 1,000 kg/m³, the oil has a density of 600 kg/m³.

306. (C) Absolute pressure is equal to the atmospheric pressure plus the hydrostatic pressure of the water. The surface area of the lake has no effect on the fluid pressure at the bottom of the lake.

$P = P_{atm} + P_{water} = 1.01 \times 10^5 \text{ Pa} + \rho g h$

$P = 1.01 \times 10^5 \text{ Pa} + (1,000 \text{ kg/m}^3)(9.8 \text{ m/s}^2)(20 \text{ m}) = 3 \times 10^5 \text{ Pa}$

The closest answer is 300,000 Pa, or 300 kPa.

A quick estimate can also be used to solve this problem. Each 10 m depth of water is approximately 1 atmosphere, so the 20 m depth of water exerts a pressure of 2 atmospheres at the bottom of the lake. The absolute, or total, pressure is therefore equal to 2 atm of water plus 1 atm of air above it, or 3 atm, which is closest to 300 kPa.

307. (A) Pressure exerted by a fluid is dependent only on the depth and density of the fluid: $P = \rho g h$. Total volume and surface area are not factors in pressure (although area can be used to determine total force: $F = PA$).

308. (C) Absolute pressure is the total pressure of all fluids above a point of reference—in this case, the pressure of water plus the pressure of the atmosphere.

$P_{abs} = P_{atm} + P_{water} = 101 \text{ kPa} + \rho g h = 1.01 \times 10^5 \text{ Pa} + (1,000 \text{ kg/m}^3)(9.8 \text{ m/s}^2)(6 \text{ m})$
$= 161,000 \text{ Pa}$

The area of the bottom of the tank is not a factor in the determination of pressure.

309. (D) First, the absolute pressure on the bottom of the tank is determined. Absolute pressure is the total pressure of all fluids above a point of reference—in this case, the pressure of water plus the pressure of the atmosphere.

$P_{abs} = P_{atm} + P_{water} = 101 \text{ kPa} + \rho g h = 1.01 \times 10^5 \text{ Pa} + (1,000 \text{ kg/m}^3)(9.8 \text{ m/s}^2)(6 \text{ m})$
$= 161,000 \text{ Pa}$

Then, the fluid force is determined using the relationship between force, pressure, and area.

$P = \dfrac{F}{A}$

$F = PA = (161,000 \text{ Pa})(50 \text{ m}^2) = 8,050,000 \text{ N}$

Hint: This multiplication is easy without a calculator: multiply the pressure by 100, then divide by 2.

310. (C) Assuming that air pressure is a small factor, the pressure due to sea water at that great depth is calculated, then force is determined by multiplying pressure by area.

$F = PA = \rho g h A = (1,025 \text{ kg/m}^3)(9.8 \text{ m/s}^2)(4,000 \text{ m})(1 \text{ m}^2) = 40,180,000 \text{ N}$

311. (D) The total fluid pressure at the bottom of a lake is equal to the sum of the atmospheric pressure and the pressure of the water. Absolute pressure at a given depth depends only on density, depth, and the value of g: $P_{abs} = P_{atm} + \rho g h$.

312. (C) The total pressure on the bubble at a depth of 21 m is approximately 3 atmospheres. (Each depth of 10 m of water exerts a pressure of about 1 atmosphere, so the total is about 2 atmospheres of water plus 1 atmosphere of air.) When the bubble reaches the surface, it has only 1 atmosphere of pressure on it. When the pressure is reduced to one third, the bubble will expand to 3 times its original volume.

313. (C) Since there is no atmosphere on the surface of the moon, there will be no buoyant force on the balloon. With only a gravitational force, the balloon will sink, regardless of changes in volume or density.

314. (D) For water and most fluids, viscosity increases as temperature decreases. An increase in viscosity means that there are more intermolecular forces, which decreases the rate at which the molecules of the fluid can move past each other and therefore decreases flow rate.

315. (C) Since all other measurements are the same, the velocities are the ratios of difference in density (squared) over viscosity.

For water: $\dfrac{(\Delta\rho)^2}{\eta} = \dfrac{(7,500 - 1,000)^2}{0.001}$

For oil: $\dfrac{(\Delta\rho)^2}{\eta} = \dfrac{(7,500 - 900)^2}{0.1}$

Since the numerators are close in value, the ratio of water to olive oil can be estimated as the inverse of velocity, or about 100 to 1.

316. (D) First, the speed of the water as it flows into the smaller pipe is determined by using the continuity equation (conservation of mass). Then, the new speed as the pipe turns to the higher level is determined by using Bernoulli's equation (conservation of energy).

(1) $A_1 v_1 = A_2 v_2$

$\pi r_1^2 v_1 = \pi r_2^2 v_2$

$(0.1 \text{ m})^2 (4 \text{ m/s}) = (0.05 \text{ m})^2 v_2$

$v_2 = \dfrac{(0.1)^2(4)}{(0.05)^2} = 16 \text{ m/s}$

(2) $\frac{1}{2}\rho v_L^2 = \frac{1}{2}\rho v_H^2 + \rho g h$

$\frac{1}{2}(16 \text{ m/s})^2 = \frac{1}{2}v_H^2 + (9.8 \text{ m/s}^2)(2.0 \text{ m})$

$128 = \frac{1}{2}v_H^2 + 20$

$v_H = \sqrt{(2)(108)}$, or about 15 m/s

Hint: Since flow rate in a pipe is inversely proportional to its area (and area is proportional to the square of the radius), doubling the diameter of a pipe quadruples the area and cuts the fluid speed to one fourth.

317. (C) When your thumb decreases the cross-sectional area of the opening of the hose, the speed of water flow must increase to conserve the mass rate of flow—a statement of the continuity equation, $A_1v_1 = A_2v_2$. However, the amount of water flowing out of the hose each second must remain constant to conserve the mass rate of flow.

318. (B) The following formula is used, where A is cross-sectional area ($\pi r^2/2$ in this case, since the semicircular area is one half the circular area and the trough is full of water) and v is the speed of water flow.

$$\frac{V}{t} = Av$$

The product of area and speed will give volume, V, per unit of time, t. For this semicircular shape, the depth at the center is the radius, r. The values in the choices are spread out enough that an estimate for the calculation will yield the correct answer.

$$V = Avt = (\tfrac{1}{2}\pi r^2)(vt) = \tfrac{1}{2}\pi(0.2 \text{ m})^2(3 \text{ m/s})(3600 \text{ s}) = 680 \text{ m}^3$$

To have the sense of how much water this is: Each cubic meter is 1,000 liters, so the flow is 680,000 liters, or about 180,000 gallons.

319. (D) Turbulence in fluid flow is defined by the Reynolds number, which is directly proportional to the density of the fluid (ρ), the diameter of the obstacle encountered or the diameter of the pipe in which the fluid flows (D), and the velocity of the fluid (v); it is inversely proportional to the viscosity of the fluid. A higher Reynolds number indicates a greater likelihood that flow will be turbulent.

320. (A) Turbulence in fluid flow is defined by the Reynolds number, which is directly proportional to the density of the fluid (ρ), the diameter of the obstacle encountered or the diameter of the pipe in which the fluid flows (D), and the velocity of the fluid (v); it is inversely proportional to the viscosity of the fluid. As the Reynolds number increases, the fluid flow is more likely to become turbulent. The sudden increase in diameter as blood flows from a small vessel into a larger one can cause turbulence.

321. (B) Both viscosity and surface tension are properties of real fluids that are not found in ideal fluids. Assumptions made about ideal fluids include no frictional losses and no interactions between molecules. Viscosity arises in fluids due to friction between the moving fluid and a surface, and surface tension is due to attractive forces among the molecules of the fluid at its surface. Density is a property of both real and ideal fluids.

322. (B) Adding an inorganic salt would actually increase surface tension in water. Heating water decreases surface tension. Adding sugar has little or no effect on surface tension. Adding a surfactant decreases surface tension.

323. (A) Using Bernoulli's equation, it is assumed that the air pressure inside the container is approximately the same as the air pressure outside the container. Since there is no water flow to speak of inside the container and no water pressure outside, these terms are canceled.

$$P_{in} + \rho gh_{in} + \tfrac{1}{2}\rho v_{in}^2 = P_{out} + \rho gh_{out} + \tfrac{1}{2}\rho v_{out}^2$$

$$\rho gh_{in} = \tfrac{1}{2}\rho v_{out}^2$$

$$(9.8 \text{ m/s}^2)(0.45 \text{ m}) = \tfrac{1}{2}v^2$$

$$v = 3.0 \text{ m/s}$$

324. (D) First, Bernoulli's equation is used to determine the pressure difference between the upper and lower surfaces of the airfoil. Then, the equation $P = F/A$ is used with the area of the airfoil to determine the force. Since the pressure below the airfoil is greater than the pressure above, the force is a "lift" force. In using Bernoulli's equation, it is assumed that the atmospheric pressure (ρgh) above and below the foil is not significantly different, so it can be canceled. The density of air is 1.29 kg/m^3.

(1) $P_{below} + \rho gh_{below} + \tfrac{1}{2}\rho v_{below}^2 = P_{above} + \rho gh_{above} + \tfrac{1}{2}\rho v_{above}^2$

$P_{below} + \tfrac{1}{2}\rho v_{below}^2 = P_{above} + \tfrac{1}{2}\rho v_{above}^2$

$P_{below} - P_{above} = \Delta P = \tfrac{1}{2}\rho v_{above}^2 - \tfrac{1}{2}\rho v_{below}^2$

$\Delta P = \tfrac{1}{2}(1.29 \text{ kg/m}^3)(50 \text{ m/s})^2 - \tfrac{1}{2}(1.29 \text{ kg/m}^3)(40 \text{ m/s})^2 = 580 \text{ Pa}$

(2) $P = \dfrac{F}{A}$

$F = PA = (580)(30) = 17{,}400 \text{ N}$

Note that the pressure in the fluid flow is lower when the speed is higher, and the pressure is higher when the speed is lower. Airfoils are designed so that air flows faster over the top, causing lower pressure on the top and higher pressure under the airfoil, thereby creating a pressure difference and a lift force.

325. (C) In applying Bernoulli's equation, it is assumed that the kinetic energy of the fluid emerging from the hose ($\tfrac{1}{2}\rho v^2$) is equal to the potential energy of the fluid (ρgh) when the water reaches maximum height. The individual water droplets behave like any small objects thrown into the air with a speed v.

$$\tfrac{1}{2}\rho v^2 = \rho gh$$

$$v = \sqrt{2gh} = \sqrt{(2)(9.8 \text{ m/s}^2)(2 \text{ m})} = 6 \text{ m/s}$$

326. (C) Bernoulli's equation is a statement of conservation of energy in fluid flow. This is easily proved by multiplying each term in the equation by volume and examining the units on each term.

$$P + \rho gh + \tfrac{1}{2}\rho v^2 = \text{constant}$$

$$PV + (\rho V)gh + \tfrac{1}{2}(\rho V)v^2 = \text{constant}$$

$$W + mgh + \tfrac{1}{2}mv^2 = \text{constant}$$

Since density times volume equals mass and pressure times volume equals work, those substitutions have been made, which reduces Bernoulli's equation to the work-energy theorem.

327. (D) First, the speed of air flow in the narrow tube is determined using the continuity equation ($A_1v_1 = A_2v_2$). Since the radius is halved and area depends on radius squared, the new area is one fourth as large, so the air speed is four times as much, or 8 m/s. Also, since the air flow is horizontal, the ρgh terms in Bernoulli's equation can be ignored.

$$P_1 + \rho gh_1 + \tfrac{1}{2}\rho v_1^2 = P_2 + \rho gh_2 + \tfrac{1}{2}\rho v_2^2$$
$$P_1 + \tfrac{1}{2}\rho v_1^2 = P_2 + \tfrac{1}{2}\rho v_2^2$$
$$P_1 - P_2 = \Delta P = \tfrac{1}{2}\rho v_2^2 - \tfrac{1}{2}\rho v_1^2$$
$$\Delta P = \tfrac{1}{2}(1.29 \text{ kg/m}^3)[(8 \text{ m/s})^2 - (2 \text{ m/s})^2] = \tfrac{1}{2}(\tfrac{4}{3})(60) = 40 \text{ Pa}$$

328. (B) Stress is the force applied to an object over a given area (F/A), and strain is the amount that the object is deformed (compressed, stretched, or bent). Strain is proportional to stress until the elastic limit is reached. Beyond the elastic limit, the object does not return to its original shape. When the stress is greater than the elastic limit, the object is permanently deformed, such as a spring that has had too much force applied to it so that it does not return to its original shape.

329. (D) The elastic limit is the value of the stress (F/A in pascals) that produces a deformation of the object such that the object does not return to its original shape. This is usually beyond the point on the plot where the stress/strain relationship ceases to be linear. Young's modulus for brass (Y) is 9×10^{10} N/m^2, so that is the slope until the stress reaches a value of about 45×10^6 Pa, which is the elastic limit. Beyond the elastic limit, the object undergoes nonelastic deformation, which can be observed as the graph begins to curve, just beyond 45 MPa. The strain, which is $\Delta L/L_o$, is a ratio that either does not have units or is expressed as a percentage.

$$\frac{F}{A} = \frac{Y\Delta L}{L_o}$$

330. (A) The shear modulus, which is the largest value, describes the amount of force required to bend or twist the bone a given amount per unit of cross-sectional area. The tension Young's modulus describes the amount of force required to stretch the bone a given amount per unit of cross-sectional area. The compression Young's modulus describes the amount of force required to compress the bone a given amount per unit of cross-sectional area. Consequently, it is easier to compress a bone than to stretch or bend (twist) it.

331. (A) The amount of stretch, or deformation, for a given force applied to a rod is derived from the Young's modulus equation, where the weight on the rod is F, Young's modulus is Y, the deformation is ΔY, the cross-sectional area is A, and the rod length is L_o.

$$\frac{F}{A} = \frac{Y\Delta L}{L_o}$$

Doubling the diameter of the rod would double the radius. Since area is proportional to radius squared, doubling the diameter would quadruple the area, meaning the deformation per unit length of rod would remain constant.

Chapter 10: Electrostatics

332. **(A)** Each electron has a charge of 1.6×10^{-19} C. This charge per electron times the number of electrons equals the total charge on the balloon.

$$\frac{\text{Total charge}}{\text{Charge per electron}} = \text{Number of electrons}$$

$$\frac{1.6 \times 10^{-8}}{1.6 \times 10^{-19}} = 1 \times 10^{11}$$

333. **(C)** When the spheres come into contact, the charge is distributed evenly across both spheres. After positive and negative charges cancel, the net charge is $-2Q$, with half of that charge on each sphere, since they are identical in size. When they are separated, each sphere then has a net charge of $-Q$.

334. **(A)** The key is that the first rod did not touch the second rod. While the negatively charged rod was near the second rod, a polarization of charge in the second rod occurred—meaning that the charge in the rod separated. Electrons moved to the end of the rod farthest from the first rod, leaving the end nearest the first rod with a positive charge. Thus, the positive end of the second rod was attracted to the negatively charged rod. However, when the negatively charged rod was removed, the charge in the second rod was redistributed and the net charge on the second rod was neutral.

335. **(B)** The key is that the first rod did not touch the second rod and was held in position while the ground wire was cut. While the negatively charged rod was near the second rod, a polarization of charge in the second rod occurred—meaning that the charge in the rod separated. Electrons moved to the end of the rod farthest from the first rod and then to the ground, leaving the second rod with a positive charge. Since the negatively charged rod was held near the second rod while the ground wire was cut, the separation of charge was maintained, so the second rod was left with a positive net charge.

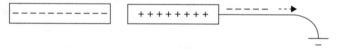

336. **(B)** Since the sphere is made of a conducting material, charges can move easily. The excess charges will repel and move to the outer surface of the sphere, distributing evenly over the surface. The insulating stand is nonconductive, so the charges are not able to move to the ground.

337. **(C)** Since the sphere is nonconducting, the negative charge transferred to the sphere remains in place at the point of contact with the rod.

338. (D) Using Coulomb's law, doubling each charge means that the electric force that each charged object exerts on the other is four times greater.

$$F_E = \frac{kq_1q_2}{R^2} = \left(\frac{1}{4\pi\varepsilon_o}\right)\left(\frac{q_1q_2}{R^2}\right)$$

$$4F_E = \frac{kq_1q_2}{R^2} = \left(\frac{1}{4\pi\varepsilon_o}\right)\left(\frac{(2q_1)(2q_2)}{R^2}\right)$$

339. (A) Using Coulomb's law, multiplying the distance between the charged objects by 4 means that the electric force that each charged object exerts on the other is one sixteenth as great. This is an application of the inverse square law: if the objects are four times farther apart, the force is $\frac{1}{4}^2$, or $\frac{1}{16}$.

$$F_E = \frac{kq_1q_2}{R^2} = \left(\frac{1}{4\pi\varepsilon_o}\right)\left(\frac{q_1q_2}{R^2}\right)$$

$$\frac{F_E}{16} = \frac{kq_1q_2}{R^2} = \left(\frac{1}{4\pi\varepsilon_o}\right)\left(\frac{q_1q_2}{(4R)^2}\right)$$

340. (D) Each of the four particles exerts the same attractive force on the electron. Due to the symmetry of the arrangement, the four force vectors effectively cancel each other, so there is no net force on the electron.

341. (A) The net electric force on q_2 is the sum of the force of q_1 on q_2, which is to the left, since the positive particle will attract the negative particle, and the force of q_3 on q_2, which is also to the left, since the negative particles repel. The magnitudes of the two forces, since they are both to the left, are added. The calculation is made easier by the 1 m distances between charges.

$$\Sigma F_E = \frac{kq_1q_2}{R^2} + \frac{kq_3q_2}{R^2} = \frac{(9 \times 10^9 \text{ N·m}^2/\text{C}^2)(2)q_1q_2}{(1 \text{ m})^2} + \frac{(9 \times 10^9 \text{ N·m}^2/\text{C}^2)(4)q_3q_2}{(1 \text{ m})^2}$$

$$= 6kq^2$$

342. (B) The electric force is the expression qE. The gravitational force (the weight (mg) of the droplet) is set equal to the electric force. The mass of the oil droplet is determined using $2e$, which stands for the charge of two electrons, for the charge, q.

$$F_G = F_E = qE$$

$$mg = qE$$

$$m = \frac{qE}{g} = \frac{2eE}{g}$$

343. (A) The symmetry of the situation should be recognized. Since the charges on the x axis are located equidistant from the y axis, they are also equidistant from point P. The electric field vectors are outward from each charge on the x axis, since they exert forces of repulsion on the charge at point P and on each other. The vectors important at point P are shown in the illustration.

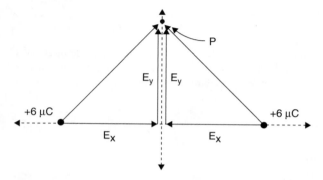

The symmetry of the x and y components of the electric field vectors should be recognized. The x components are equal in magnitude and opposite in direction, so they cancel. Thus, the only effective electric field vectors at point P due to the charged particles on the x axis are the y components. These y components are equal in both magnitude and direction, so one of the y components can be calculated, then doubled, to determine the answer.

$$F = \left(\frac{1}{4\pi\varepsilon_o}\right)\left(\frac{Q^2}{R^2}\right) = \frac{kQ^2}{R^2} = \frac{(9 \times 10^9 \text{ N·m}^2/\text{C}^2)(6 \times 10^{-6}\text{C})^2}{(3\sqrt{2} \text{ m})^2}$$

$$F_y = F\sin 45° = F\frac{\sqrt{2}}{2} = \left(\frac{(9 \times 10^9 \text{ N·m}^2/\text{C}^2)(6 \times 10^{-6} \text{ C})^2}{(3\sqrt{2} \text{ m})^2}\right)\left(\frac{\sqrt{2}}{2}\right)$$

$$2F_y = (2)\left(\frac{(9 \times 10^9 \text{ N·m}^2/\text{C}^2)(6 \times 10^{-6} \text{ C})^2}{(3\sqrt{2} \text{ m})^2}\right)\left(\frac{\sqrt{2}}{2}\right) = \frac{18\sqrt{2}}{2} \times 10^{-3} = (3)(0.7)(10^{-3})$$
$$= 0.025 \text{ N}$$

344. (D) The electric force of the proton on the electron is equal to and in the opposite direction of the force of the electron on the proton. The force is calculated using Coulomb's law. The charge on the proton is the same as the charge on the electron.

$$F = \left(\frac{1}{4\pi\varepsilon_o}\right)\left(\frac{Q^2}{R^2}\right) = \frac{kQ^2}{R^2} = \frac{(9 \times 10^9 \text{ N·m}^2/\text{C}^2)(1.6 \times 10^{-19} \text{ C})^2}{(1.59 \times 10^{-11} \text{ m})^2} = 9.1 \times 10^{-7} \text{ N}$$

Note: The correct answer could also be determined by using powers of ten.

345. (D) The electric force of the 12 protons in the nucleus on the electron is equal to and in the opposite direction of the force of the electron on the protons. The force is calculated using Coulomb's law. The charge on each proton is the same as the charge on the electron.

$$F = \left(\frac{1}{4\pi\varepsilon_o}\right)\left(\frac{Q^2}{R^2}\right) = \frac{kQ^2}{R^2} = \frac{(9 \times 10^9 \text{ N·m}^2/\text{C}^2)(12)(1.6 \times 10^{-19} \text{ C})^2}{(70 \times 10^{-12} \text{ m})^2} = 5.6 \times 10^{-7} \text{ N}$$

Note: The correct answer could also be determined by using powers of ten.

346. (C) The symmetry of the situation should be recognized. Since the charges on the x axis are located equidistant from the y axis, they are also equidistant from point P. The electric field vectors are outward from each charge on the x axis, and the only electric field vectors important at point P are shown in the illustration.

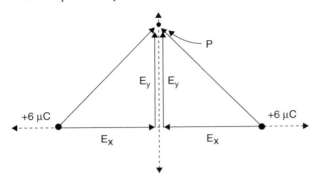

The symmetry of the x and y components of the electric field vectors should be recognized. The x components are equal in magnitude and opposite in direction, so they cancel. Thus, the only effective electric field vectors at point P due to the charged particles on the x axis are the y components. These y components are equal in both magnitude and direction, so one of the y components can be calculated, then doubled, to determine the answer.

$$E = \left(\frac{1}{4\pi\varepsilon_o}\right)\left(\frac{Q}{R^2}\right) = \frac{kQ}{R^2} = \frac{(9 \times 10^9 \text{ N·m}^2/\text{C}^2)(6 \times 10^{-6} \text{ C})}{(3\sqrt{2} \text{ m})^2}$$

$$E_y = E \sin 45° = E\frac{\sqrt{2}}{2} = \left(\frac{(9 \times 10^9 \text{ N·m}^2/\text{C}^2)(6 \times 10^{-6} \text{ C})}{(3\sqrt{2} \text{ m})^2}\right)\left(\frac{\sqrt{2}}{2}\right)$$

$$2E_y = (2)\left(\frac{(9 \times 10^9 \text{ N·m}^2/\text{C}^2)(6 \times 10^{-6} \text{ C})}{(3\sqrt{2} \text{ m})^2}\right)\left(\frac{\sqrt{2}}{2}\right) = \frac{6\sqrt{2}}{2} \times 10^3 = 4.2 \times 10^3 \text{ N/C}$$

347. (C) The following equation is used.

$$E = \left(\frac{1}{4\pi\varepsilon_o}\right)\left(\frac{Q}{R^2}\right) = \frac{kQ}{R^2} = \frac{(9 \times 10^9 \text{ N·m}^2/\text{C}^2)(2 \times 10^{-9} \text{ C})}{(0.02 \text{ m})^2} = 4.5 \times 10^4 \text{ N/C}$$

348. (D) The electric field, which is outward from a positively charged particle, is directed toward the center from each of the four particles. Since the charge of each particle is the same and each particle is the same distance from the center, the vectors effectively cancel each other, creating a net electric field of zero at the center of the square. Thus, any charged particle placed at the center of the square would have no electric force exerted on it, since $F = qE$.

349. (D) The net effect for this arrangement is zero, since the field vectors at the center due to the positive charges are equal in magnitude and opposite in direction; those two vectors cancel. The same is true for the two negative charges. This type of arrangement has symmetry, and it is helpful to look for symmetry when examining any situation. In this instance, symmetry involves vectors that cancel each other.

350. (C) Once the metal surface of the sphere is charged, all charges are mobile and repel each other, so once equilibrium is established, the charges will distribute evenly on the outer surface of the sphere. All electric field vectors due to the charges will cancel inside the sphere, so there will be no electric field inside the sphere. (It is helpful to remember that the electric field inside any conductor is zero.) The strongest field, then, is just outside the sphere, becoming weaker as the distance from the sphere increases.

351. (B) The electric field will exert a force on positive charges, moving them to the right side of the sphere: $F = qE$. This will leave the right side more positive and the left side more negative. Even if the field were strong enough to remove electrons, they would not move to the right, so choice (D) is not correct.

352. (C) When the sphere is placed into the field, the field will exert a force on charges within the sphere, separating and polarizing the charges so that the right side of the sphere will be more positive and the left side will be more negative. This concentration of charges increases the field on both left and right, altering the field so that it will be stronger in those regions (and there is a higher density of field lines on the left and right). However, there will be no electric field within the sphere.

353. (D) All statements are true except (D). Since the charge is uniform on both plates, the electric field between the plates is constant. It is the electric potential that increases from the bottom to the top.

354. (D) The net electric field at point P is the vector sum of the field vector to the right from charged particle 1 and the field vector to the right due to negative-charged particle 2. The magnitudes of the field vectors are added, because they are both to the right. The calculation is made easier by the 1 m distance between the charges.

$$\Sigma E = \frac{kq_1}{r^2} + \frac{kq_2}{r^2} = \frac{k(q)}{l^2} + \frac{k(2q)}{l^2} = 3kq$$

355. (D) The potential energy of two electric charges is equal to kQq/r. The amount of work to assemble the group of charges would be equal to the sum of the potential energies of each pair of charges, taken two at a time. For the three positive charges, three positive potential energies would be added. For the three negative charges, the same three quantities would be added, since the product of the two negative charges in each term would be positive. The amount of work in both cases would be the same. For the two positive charges and one negative charge, one positive term and two negative terms, all of equal magnitude, would be added, so the net work would be less than in the first two cases. (For two negative charges and one positive charge, one positive term and two negative terms, all of equal magnitude, would be added.)

356. (C) Electric field is inversely proportional to distance squared, but electric potential is inversely proportional to distance; the formula for each follows.

$$E = \frac{kQ}{R^2}$$

$$V = \frac{kQ}{R}$$

357. (D) Electric potential is defined by the equation $V = kQ/r$, so potential varies inversely with distance, but does not follow the inverse square law. The quantities in all other choices have distance squared in the denominator. For example, as the distance from the source is doubled, the magnitude of the quantity decreases to one quarter. If the distance is tripled, the quantity decreases to one ninth, and so on.

358. (B) Electric potential is a scalar quantity that is directly proportional to charge: $V = kQ/r$. Positive and negative values of potential simply add numerically. Since the $-4q$ charge is twice as large, it should be twice as far from the zero point as the $2q$ charge. At $x = 4$, the potential from the negative charge is $-4kQ/2$, or $-2kQ$. At $x = 4$, the potential from the $2q$ charge is $2kQ/1$, or $+2kQ$. These values add to zero at $x = 4$.

359. (B) Electric potential energy, U, is the product of charge, q, and electric potential difference, ΔV, from the definition of electric potential difference.

$$\Delta V = \frac{U}{q}$$

The answer in joules is the product of charge in coulombs and potential difference in volts. One volt equals one joule per coulomb.

$$\Delta U = q\Delta V = (0.5\ \text{C})(1.5\ \text{V}) = 0.75\ \text{J}$$

360. (C) The magnitude of the change in electric potential is equal to Ed, from the equation $E = -\Delta V/\Delta d$, which does not depend on the magnitude of the charge. The path is measured along the direction of the field, using the component of the 0.02 m distance in the direction of the field.

$$V = (100)(0.02) \cos 60°$$

361. (D) A line drawn so that every point on the line has the same electric potential due to the three charges would be an equipotential line. The sum of the electric potentials due to the three charges would have to be the same at every point on the line.

$$\sum_{n=3} \frac{kQq}{r} = \text{constant}$$

Equipotential lines are perpendicular to the electric field. For three positive charges, the equipotential line would be a curved shape surrounding the three charges.

362. (D) An equipotential line for both charged particles is a set of points all of which have the same potential, determined by adding the potentials due to each of the charges.

$$\Sigma V = \frac{kq}{r_1} + \frac{kq}{r_2} = kq\left(\frac{1}{r_1} + \frac{1}{r_2}\right)$$

Inspection reveals cases for each of the three lines where the contribution due to one charge remains fairly constant while the contribution due to the other charge changes, causing varying values for the sum of the potentials.

363. (A) The calculation involves only multiplication and operations with exponents.

$$U = \frac{kq_1q_2}{r} = \left(\frac{1}{4\pi\varepsilon_o}\right)\left(\frac{q_1q_2}{r}\right)$$

$$U = \frac{(9 \times 10^9)(3 \times 10^{-6})(3 \times 10^{-6})}{1 \times 10^{-2}} = 81 \times 10^{-1} = 8.1\,\text{J}$$

Common mistakes are to square the distance, r, producing the incorrect answer in choice (C), and to use only one of the charges, producing the incorrect answer in choice (D). The incorrect answer in choice (B) results from an incorrect operation with exponents.

364. (A) An electric field, E, exerts a force on the positive charge, q, so that the force is in the same direction as the field, and a negative charge has a force exerted on it in the opposite direction of the field: $F = qE$. Thus, an electric dipole will align so that the positive end is to the right. In any other orientation, such as perpendicular to the field, there will be an electric force that causes the dipole to rotate. The dipole remains stationary once it is aligned with the positive end to the right, because the forces on the positive and negative regions of the dipole are equal in magnitude but opposite in direction, so there would be no net force in this position.

Another approach to this problem recognizes that the dipole itself has an electric field, with field lines extending outward from the positive end (to the left from the left end of the dipole) and inward toward the negative end (to the left into the right end of the dipole). The dipole will then align itself in the electric field so that the field lines align.

365. (C) Water exhibits its unique properties due to hydrogen bonding, which causes, for example, ice to float in water. Hydrogen bonding occurs because of the structure of a water molecule—with the two hydrogen atoms located on one side of the molecule and the oxygen atom on the other side.

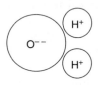

The hydrogen end of the molecule is more positive, and the oxygen end is more negative, making the water molecule a common electric dipole. A magnet and Earth are magnetic dipoles, and a proton is considered an electric monopole, since it is entirely positive.

366. (C) The calculation of charge enclosed for this symmetrical shape is simple. The Gaussian surface defines the charge enclosed. Since this is a conductive sphere, the positive charge will move to the outside surface of the sphere, once equilibrium is established, since the positive charges repel each other and can be conducted as far as possible from each other on the sphere. Gaussian surface A encloses the sphere and so will enclose the charge Q; however, Gaussian surface B is inside the sphere, where there is no charge.

367. (A) Electric flux, Φ, is the product of the electric field and the area in a given direction. Since the electric field is entirely in the x direction, there would be no flux in the y or z direction. In the x direction, the flux into the left side of the cube is $E \cdot A$, or (100 N/C)(4 m²). However, the flux is the same out of the right side of the cube, so the *net* flux through the cube is zero. Note: The net flux through the cube is proportional to the electric charge enclosed by the cube, which is zero, since the cube is uncharged.

368. (B) The question doesn't ask for the flux in any other direction, so only the flux through the right and left sides of the cube must be considered. The flux through the left side of the cube is due to the electric field: $\Phi = E \cdot A$. Since the flux through the left side of the cube is only one half that, it might be assumed that a negative charge in the cube would create a field inward, canceling part of the electric field outward on the right side.

Chapter 11: Electric Circuits

369. (A) Current is the rate of flow of charge, so $I = \Delta Q / \Delta t = (3.6 \times 10^{-6})/(10 \times 10^{-3}) = 3.6 \times 10^{-4}$ A, or 0.36×10^{-3} A, which is 0.36 mA.

370. (A) By definition, current is the rate of flow of charge ($I = \Delta Q / \Delta t$). If current is in amps, charge is in coulombs, and time is in seconds, then 1 amp is equal to 1 coulomb per second.

371. (B) First, the equivalent resistance, or total resistance of the two resistors, is determined. Since there are only two resistors in parallel, this can be done quickly using product over sum; the total resistance is 18/9, or 2 Ω. Using Ohm's law, $V = IR$, the current must be 10 A. Because the resistance is in a ratio of 2:1, the current will split in the same ratio, with the larger current taking the path of least resistance. The current split is two thirds of the current to the 3 Ω resistor and one third of the current to the 6 Ω resistor. Thus, the current in the 3 Ω resistor is two thirds of 10, or 6.7 A.

Another approach to the problem is to recognize that the sum of potential differences in any loop must be zero, so the potential difference is 20 V in each of the resistors. Using Ohm's law, $I = V/R = 20/3 = 6.67$ A.

372. (B) First, the equivalent resistance of the three resistors is determined. Using product over sum, the resistance of the two resistors in parallel is determined: $R^2/2R$, or ½R. Then, the resistor in series is added to find the total resistance: $R_T = R + \frac{1}{2}R = \frac{3}{2}R$. Ohm's law is used to determine current from the battery: $I = V/R_T = V/(\frac{3}{2}R) = 2V/3R$. The total current splits equally into the two parallel branches, so that the resistor on the far right gets one half of the current, or $V/3R$.

373. (D) The total resistance of the two resistors in series is 50 Ω. Ohm's law is used to determine current: $I = V/R = 10/50 = 0.2$ A. Since the resistors are in series, all the current flows through each resistor. Ohm's law is used again, this time to determine potential difference: $V = IR = (0.2$ A$)(20$ Ω$) = 4$ V.

Another approach to the problem is to recognize that the 10 V potential difference across the resistors is split, with part of the difference in each resistor. Since both have the same current, we know that the smaller resistor will get the smaller share of the potential difference: two fifths of 10 V equals 4 V in the 20 Ω resistor, leaving 6 V in the 30 Ω resistor.

374. (B) Applying Kirchhoff's loop rule, the sum of potential differences for all elements in the circuit will be zero: $\varepsilon - IR - Ir = 0$. In this case, $\varepsilon = 12$ V, I is the current, $R = 16$ Ω, and $r = 2$ Ω.

$12 - I(16) - I(2) = 0$

$I = 0.67$ A

375. (D) The emf of a battery, minus the electric potential difference due to the internal resistance in the battery, is the potential difference at the poles of the battery, or the voltage delivered to the external circuit: $V_{ext} = \varepsilon - Ir$.

10 V $= 12$ V $- (1\ A)(r)$

$r = 2$ Ω

376. (B) First, the equivalent resistance for the two parallel branches on the right is determined. In those branches, the two bulbs in series on the far right have a resistance of 200 Ω, which is in parallel with 100 Ω. Using product over sum, the equivalent in parallel is 20,000/300, or 67 Ω. Next, the two bulbs on the left are in series with the parallel branches, so these are added to the resistance of the other three bulbs. The total resistance is $100 + 100 + 67 = 267$ Ω.

377. (C) The equivalent (total) resistance is the size of one resistor that could replace the combination of resistors and still deliver the same current and power to the external circuit. Product over sum is used to determine the equivalent resistance of the two resistors in parallel at the right: $100^2/200$, or 50 Ω. Since the third resistor is in series with the parallel combination, its resistance is added, for a total of 150 Ω.

378. (D) The parallel rule for addition of resistors in parallel can be used to determine the resistance of the two resistors in parallel at the bottom, but the quickest method is to use product over sum: $40^2/80$, or 20 Ω. This resistance is added to the resistances of the other two resistors, which are in series with this combination. The total resistance is $20 + 20 + 20$, or 60 Ω.

379. (B) There is no mention that the resistors are equal to each other, so it cannot be assumed that the current splits equally in the branches. However, by Kirchhoff's loop rule (conservation of energy), the potential difference across each branch must be the same. In fact, as more resistors are added in parallel, the total resistance decreases.

380. (B) The resistance of a resistor is directly proportional to the product of resistivity and length, and inversely proportional to cross-sectional area.

$$R = \frac{\rho L}{A}$$

Choice (B) states this formula in terms of ρ. In applying this formula, R is in ohms (Ω), ρ is in ohm-meters, L is in meters, and A is in square meters.

381. (A) It is true that an electric potential difference (or voltage)—applied by a battery or power supply to each end of a wire—will result in an electric field in the wire, which will cause electrons to move from one end of the wire to the other ($F = qE$). Choice (B) is not correct, because electrical conductivity is a property of the material—not the size of the wire. For example, copper has high conductivity because even a small electric field causes a large current to flow in the wire. A material like plastic has low conductivity (and high resistivity). Choice (C) is not correct, because increasing the cross-sectional area of a wire decreases resistance. (This is analogous to a water pipe, where water flows at a greater rate in a larger pipe.)

382. (D) The energy stored in a capacitor, C, is equal to $\frac{1}{2}CV^2$, where C is capacitance in farads (F) and V is electric potential difference in volts (V). If the potential difference, V, is one half as much in the second case, the energy will be one fourth of 100 µJ, or 25 µJ.

383. (B) The energy stored in a capacitor, C, is equal to $\frac{1}{2}CV^2$. The prefix *micro-* (μ) means 10^{-6}.

$$U_C = \frac{1}{2}CV^2 = \frac{1}{2}(2000 \times 10^{-6} \text{ F})(10 \text{ V})^2 = 0.1 \text{ J}$$

Choices (C) and (D) are distractors for those who forget to incorporate the prefix μ in their calculations.

384. (A) With all other relevant factors remaining constant, doubling the distance between the plates requires work, since the plates have opposite charges and attract each other.

385. (D) Since $U_C = \frac{1}{2}CV^2$, doubling the potential difference on the capacitor would quadruple the energy stored in the capacitor.

386. (A) Charge is conserved here in much the same way that current must be the same in all parts of a series circuit with resistors. The charge on each capacitor is the same. Since $Q = C/V$, the potential difference on each capacitor is inversely proportional to the capacitance. Therefore, the smaller capacitor has twice the potential difference. By Kirchhoff's loop rule, the smaller capacitor has a 6.7 V potential difference and the larger capacitor has a 3.3 V potential difference.

387. (A) The total capacitance for two capacitors in series is calculated in the opposite way that resistors in series are added. The product over sum method (or reciprocal addition rule for just two components) is used.

$$C_T = \frac{(2000 \times 10^{-6})(4000 \times 10^{-6})}{(2000 \times 10^{-6}) + (4000 \times 10^{-6})} = \frac{8 \times 10^{-6}}{6000 \times 10^{-6}} = 1300 \text{ µF}$$

388. (A) The total capacitance for two capacitors in parallel is calculated in the opposite way that resistors in parallel are added. The capacitance for capacitors in parallel are added, so the equivalent capacitance is 6,000 μF.

389. (D) The capacitance changes when the dielectric constant (κ) is changed.

$$C = \frac{\kappa A}{d}$$

When the dielectric constant is one half as much, the capacitance is reduced to one half. Using the equation $Q = CV$, the charge on the capacitor will then be one half, since the voltage is the same in both cases.

390. (D) After a very long time, the capacitor is completely charged, so no more current flows through the resistor. With no current in the resistor, there is no potential difference (V) in the resistor (R), due to Ohm's law, $V = IR$. Therefore, by Kirchhoff's loop rule, the sum of voltage changes around the loop must be zero, and the voltage on the capacitor, V_C, must be the same as the emf. It is known that $V_C = 20$ V and $C = 1,000$ μF. Q can be determined by using the equation $Q = CV$: $Q = (1,000 \text{ μF})(20 \text{ V}) = 20,000$ μC. The resistance has no effect on the final charge in this circuit; adding a resistor only slows the charging rate.

391. (C) After a long time, it can be assumed that the capacitor is completely charged, so no more current moves in that branch of the circuit. However, the current still flows in the large loop that includes the two resistors. It is necessary to find the potential difference across the bottom resistor in the diagram so that the potential difference across the capacitor can be calculated. The total resistance of the two resistors (which are now in series with each other) is 100 Ω. Using Ohm's law ($V = IR$), the current in the resistors is $I = V/R = 10/100 = 0.1$ A. Then, the potential difference in the bottom resistor is calculated, again using Ohm's law: $V = IR = (0.1 \text{ A})(50 \text{ Ω}) = 5$ V. Using Kirchhoff's loop rule on the small loop on the left, the sum of voltages must equal zero. (Even though there is no current flowing in the branch that contains the capacitor, there is still a voltage drop across the capacitor.)

$$\varepsilon - V_C - V_R = 0$$
$$10 - V_C - 5 = 0$$
$$V_C = 5 \text{ V}$$

392. (A) In choice (A), the power is equal to change in potential energy divided by time ($mgh/t = 100/2 = 50$ W). In choice (B), the power is equal to average force times average velocity ($P = Fv = 30$ W). In choice (C), the power is equal to change in kinetic energy divided by time ($P = \Delta K/t = 40/20 = 2$ W). In choice (D), the power is equal to current squared times resistance ($P = I^2R = (2 \text{ A})^2(10 \text{ Ω}) = 40$ W).

393. (B) Power (P) is defined as the product of potential difference (V) and current (I). Since the question does not provide the current or ask for the current, Ohm's law is used to substitute for current in order to solve for power (in watts).

$$P = VI$$

$$V = IR \text{ and } I = \frac{V}{R}$$

$$\therefore P = \frac{V^2}{R} = \frac{(12)^2}{4} = 36 \text{ W}$$

394. (D) First, the equivalent resistance of the four resistors is determined. Product over sum is used to find the resistance of the two 40 Ω resistors in parallel: $R = 40^2/80 = 20 \ \Omega$. The resistance of the two 20 Ω resistors, which are in series with the parallel pair of resistors, is added to determine the total resistance: $R_T = 20 + 20 + 20 = 60 \ \Omega$. Since the potential difference and resistance are known, the power formula ($P = VI$) and Ohm's law ($V = IR$) are combined to obtain the total power output: $P = V^2/R = (30)^2/60 = 15$ W.

395. (D) The first three statements are true regarding alternating current circuits. The root mean square (rms) is the square of the average of the squared values, which is an average without positive or negative direction. Since $P = IV$, multiplying the rms current times the rms voltage gives a value for the power for the circuit.

396. (C) In a transformer, the alternating current (AC) in the input, or primary, coils induces an alternating current in the output, or secondary, coils. Neglecting loss to heating, power output equals power input.

$$P_{in} = P_{out}$$

$$V_{in}I_{in} = V_{out}I_{out}$$

$$(120 \text{ V})(I_{in}) = (9 \text{ V})(350 \text{ mA})$$

$$I_{in} = 26 \text{ mA}$$

This is called a "step down" transformer, because it decreases the potential difference (voltage). The ratio of the number of coils of wire in the primary coils to the number of coils of wire in the secondary coils is the ratio of input voltage to output voltage.

Chapter 12: Magnetic Fields and Electromagnetism

397. (A) Using a right-hand rule, curl the fingers of your right hand so they point in the direction in which the current is flowing in the loops (from positive to negative). Your thumb should extend to the right (the direction of the magnetic field inside the loop), since the current flows from positive to negative. Thus, the right end of the loop is a north pole and the left end of the loop is a south pole.

398. (B) The magnetic field for a coil is directly proportional to the number of turns and to the current and is inversely proportional to the radius. Both choices (B) and (C) cannot be true, so choice (D) cannot be correct. It is true that inserting an iron rod into the center of a coil will increase the magnetic field strength—a method used for electromagnets and to concentrate the magnetic field in transformers.

399. (D) Using a right-hand rule, extend your thumb in the direction of the current and curl your fingers to represent the magnetic field curved around each wire. For the top wire, the magnetic field is out of the page in region 1, into the page in region 2, and into the page in region 3. For the bottom wire, the magnetic field is into the page in region 1, into the page in region 2, and out of the page in region 3. For the net magnetic field to be zero in any of the regions, the field due to one wire must be into the page and the field due to the other wire must be out of the page. This is not possible in region 2, since both wires contribute to a magnetic field into the page, regardless of the size of the field. In region 2, they will never cancel or add to zero.

400. (B) Using a right-hand rule, extend your thumb in the direction of the current and curl your fingers to represent the magnetic field curved around each wire. For the top wire, the magnetic field is into the page at point P. For the bottom wire, the magnetic field is also into the page at point P. Therefore, the currents in both wires contribute to a net magnetic field into the page at point P.

401. (D) Using a right-hand rule, extend your thumb in the direction of the current and curl your fingers to represent the magnetic field curved around each wire. For the top wire, the magnetic field is into the page at point P. For the bottom wire, the magnetic field is out of the page at point P. If the currents are of equal magnitude and the distance from each wire to point P is the same, the currents contribute magnetic fields of equal magnitude but opposite direction, which add as vectors to zero.

$$B = \frac{\mu_o I}{2\pi R}$$

402. (C) A magnetic field exerts a force on a moving charged particle of a magnitude that depends on the size of the charge on the particle, the component of the velocity that is perpendicular to the magnetic field, and the strength of the magnetic field. In choice (A), there is no force, because the charge is not moving. In choice (B), the charged particle is moving along the field lines, so it has no velocity component perpendicular to the field, and the force is zero. Both choices (C) and (D) present situations in which the magnetic field would exert a force, but the velocity is entirely perpendicular to the magnetic field line in choice (C), so the largest force is exerted in the situation presented there.

403. (D) Inside a current-carrying coil (called a solenoid), the magnetic field is uniform, so it has the same strength at every point inside the coil. Outside the coil, the magnetic field can be considered to be zero.

404. (D) A charge at rest with respect to a uniform magnetic field will not experience a force and thus will not move, since $F_B = qv \times B$. A charge at rest in an electric field, however, will experience a force: $F_E = qE$.

405. (C) The magnetic field around a long, straight, current-carrying wire is in a circular pattern around the wire. If you extend the thumb of your right hand in the direction of the current in the wire, your curled fingers indicate the direction of the magnetic field around the wire. The magnitude of the magnetic field increases with current (I) and decreases with distance (R) from the wire.

$$B = \frac{\mu_o I}{2\pi R}$$

406. (D) Choices (A), (B), and (C) all describe Earth's magnetic field. A magnetic compass has a defined north pole, and this end of the compass needle points toward geographic north. Since a north pole is attracted to a south pole, the north end of the compass must point toward Earth's south magnetic pole, placing that pole near Earth's north geographic pole. This would mean that Earth's magnetic field lines would emerge from its north magnetic pole in Antarctica and go back into the Earth at the south magnetic pole in northern Canada. Magnetic field lines make continuous loops, and a magnetic compass needle will align itself along those lines.

407. (A) Using a right-hand rule, curl the fingers of your right hand so they point in the direction the current is flowing in the loops (from positive to negative). Your thumb should extend to the right, which is the direction of the magnetic field inside the loops. Therefore, the right end of each loop is a north pole, and the left end of each loop is a south pole. These act like magnets. Since north and south magnetic poles attract, choice (A) is the correct answer.

408. (D) The magnetic fields in materials depend on the pairing of electrons, the spin nature of electrons, and the alignment of atoms within the materials, creating magnetic domains. All of the statements in choices (A), (B), and (C) contribute to the explanation of why some materials have magnetic fields. In most materials, the opposing electron spins of paired electrons effectively cancel each other, creating no net magnetic field. In some materials, not all electrons are paired, so there is a net magnetic field. In addition, the magnetic atoms tend to align strongly with each other, magnifying the magnetic effect.

409. (C) The force on the protons as they enter the magnetic field is described by a vector cross product: $F = qv \times B$. Only the component of the velocity that crosses the field lines will produce a force. Using a right-hand rule, the index finger (representing velocity) points to the right and the other fingers (representing the B field) point down on the page, so the thumb (representing force) is into the page. (The index finger, other fingers, and thumb must all be mutually perpendicular.)

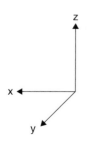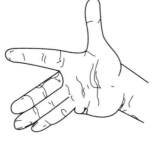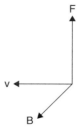

410. (C) The centripetal force to keep the charged particle moving in a circle is provided by the magnetic force. The two expressions are set equal in order to solve for mass, m, using $2e$ for the charge, q, and noting that the particle's motion is perpendicular to the field, so maximum force is exerted on the particle.

$$F_B = qvB$$

$$F_{cent} = \frac{mv^2}{R}$$

$$2evB = \frac{mv^2}{R}$$

$$m = \frac{2eBR}{v}$$

411. (C) First, the right-hand rule is used to determine the charge on the particle. If the force is down on the page in the $-y$ direction, the magnetic field is into the page in the $-z$ direction, and the velocity is to the right in the $+x$ direction, the left hand must be used, which means that the particle is negative. The negative particle has a magnetic force on it downward on the page, so there must be an electric force upward on the page in order to balance the forces so that the particle can move in a straight line. Using the equation $F = qE$, the force and electric field are in the same direction for a positive particle. For this negative particle, the force is in the opposite direction of the electric field. Therefore, for the electric force to be upward, the electric field must be downward on the page, or in the $-y$ direction.

412. (B) For the electron to move in a straight line across the page, the net force on the charge must be zero. The magnetic force on the electron is upward on the page, so the electric force should be downward on the page. However, for the electric force to be downward on the page, the electric field needs to be upward on the page, since the electric force on a negative charge is in the opposite direction as the electric field: $F = qE$. (Force on a positive charge is in the same direction as the electric field in this vector equation.) This is the "crossed fields" effect, that is, crossed electric and magnetic fields can apply equal force on a charge so that the charge moves in an undeflected path.

413. (D) Using the right-hand rule and then reversing direction for the negative charge (or using the left hand instead of the right), the magnetic force is found to be directed into the page. The electron will experience a force into the page and then continue in a circular motion in and out of the page, with the magnetic force providing the centripetal force: $F = qv \times B$.

414. (B) The charge, q, on a proton is the same as the charge on an electron, except that it is positive. This charge, which is 1.6×10^{-19} C, is often simply called e. The equation $F = qv \times B$ is applied, where q is the charge (e in this case), v is the component of the velocity that is perpendicular to the field lines ($v \sin 60°$), and B is the magnetic field.

415. (D) The right-hand rule is used to determine that if the charges were positive, they would curve outward on the page, toward the curved end of the magnet. Since these are electrons, the opposite occurs, so the electrons curve inward on the page, toward the open end of the magnet and away from the magnet. To use the right-hand rule, point your index finger in the direction of velocity, extend your other fingers perpendicular to velocity to represent the magnetic field (which is from north to south), then extend your thumb to show the direction of magnetic force. This magnetic force changes the direction of the motion of the charged particles but does not change their speed.

416. (D) Since both the wire and magnet are stationary, there is no relative motion between the electrons in the wire and the magnetic field. Therefore, there is no force from the magnetic field on the electrons and no current produced ($F = qv \times B \sin \theta = qv \times B$).

417. (C) With a greater speed, the second particle with move in a larger radius. This can be proved by setting the magnetic force on the particle equal to the centripetal force and examining the effect on speed, v.

$$F_B = F_C$$

$$qvB = \frac{mv^2}{R}$$

$$v = \frac{qBR}{m}$$

418. (B) Conventional current, I, is defined as the direction in which positive charges move, and a current-carrying wire has a magnetic field in a circular pattern around it. By using your right hand with your thumb extended in the direction of the current in the top wire, you can determine that the top wire creates a magnetic field into the page at the bottom wire. This magnetic field exerts a force on the positive charges moving to the left in the bottom wire ($F = qv \times B$). Next, use the cross-product right-hand rule to determine the direction of the force from the top wire on the bottom wire. The following illustration indicates that v is to the left, B is into the page, and the force is downward on the page. This means that the top wire repels the bottom wire. Since forces come in pairs, the bottom wire repels the top wire with the same force.

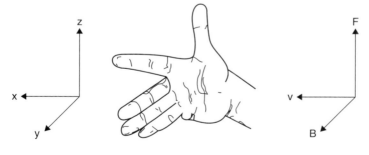

This result can be checked by considering the force the bottom wire exerts on the top wire. Using the right-hand rule, with your thumb to the left along the bottom wire, you can determine that the bottom wire creates a magnetic field into the page at the top wire. The charges in the top wire are moving to the right (since the current is to the right). Using the cross-product right-hand rule, with v to the right (your index finger), B into the page (your other fingers), and force upward on the page (your thumb), you can determine that the bottom wire also repels the top wire—so they move apart.

419. (D) The equation to use is $F_B = ILB$, where F_B is the magnetic force, I is the current in the wire, L is the length of the wire perpendicular to the magnetic field, and B is the magnetic field strength. $F_B = (0.5 \text{ A})(0.1 \text{ m})(1.5 \text{ T}) = 0.075 \text{ N}$. This equation is derived from the equation $F_B = qv \times B = qv \times B \sin \theta$, so the right-hand rule is applied similarly. Using your right hand, point your index finger in the direction of the current in length L, extend your other fingers in the direction of magnetic field B, and extend your thumb in the direction of the force on the wire, F.

Note: If the wire were not perpendicular to the magnetic field, the component that is perpendicular to the field would be used to calculate force. If the wire ran parallel to the field, there would be no magnetic force on the wire.

420. (A) If the magnetic field is increasing out of the page, then by Lenz's law, a current will be induced in the loop to oppose the change that the magnetic field is producing. Thus, the current in the loop must increase into the page. Using a right-hand rule, curl the fingers of your right hand to represent the direction of current in the loop and point your thumb in the direction of the field produced by the current in the loop. The opposing field must be into the page, so point your thumb into the page—and your fingers will curl clockwise to show the current direction in the loop.

421. (D) The magnetic field is outward from the north pole and is strongest near the pole. As the magnet drops downward toward the loop, the magnetic flux in the loop increases downward. By Lenz's law, a current will be induced in the loop that creates a magnetic field opposing the change due to the magnet. In a view from the top, a counterclockwise current in the loop would have a magnetic field upward, opposing the increasing magnetic field downward. Using a right-hand rule, curl the fingers of your right hand around the loop counterclockwise and point your thumb upward in the direction of the magnetic field created by the current in the loop.

As the magnet drops through and leaves the plane of the loop moving downward, the magnetic flux in the loop decreases downward. A current in the loop is created to oppose this by increasing the magnetic field downward. An increase in the magnetic field downward would be created by a clockwise current in the loop. Point the thumb of your right hand downward, so that your fingers curl clockwise, indicating the direction of current induced in the loop.

422. (B) One approach to this problem is to think of a positive charge located in the right edge of the loop that is moving into the field. The right-hand rule is applied to this positive charge, which is moving to the right through a magnetic field that is into the page. With your index finger pointing to the right (velocity) and your other fingers directed into the page (magnetic field), your extended thumb (force) would be upward on the page in the right side of the loop. This starts a current moving counterclockwise completely around the loop. The applicable equation is $F = qv \times B$. (Note: This method applies only if the loop is partially inside the field. If the loop were completely immersed in the field, the force on a charge on the opposite side of the loop would experience a force in the same direction, but the current direction would be in the opposite direction, so no net current would flow.)

A second approach to this problem is to apply Lenz's law. As the loop moves into the magnetic field, the magnetic flux into the page increases as more area of the loop moves into the field. This increase in flux into the page induces a current in the loop such that it creates a magnetic field to oppose the increase. The current in the loop must be counterclockwise to create an increasing magnetic field *out of* the page to oppose the increasing magnetic field *into* the page. The direction of the induced current is determined by applying the "curled fingers" right-hand rule: curl your fingers in the direction of the current so that your extended thumb points out of the page to represent the direction of the magnetic field from the induced current.

423. (C) As the magnet enters the coil, the magnetic flux increases inside the coil, so a current will be induced in the coil that creates a magnetic field to oppose this increase. Then, as the magnet leaves the coil at the other end, the flux in the coil decreases, so the direction of current will reverse to create a magnetic field in the opposite direction to oppose the decrease. This is an application of Lenz's law.

424. (A) One approach to this problem is to think of a positive charge located in the left edge of the loop that is moving out of the field. The right-hand rule is applied to this positive charge, which is moving to the right through a magnetic field that is into the page. With your index finger pointing to the right (velocity) and your other fingers directed into the page (magnetic field), your extended thumb (force) would be upward on the page in the left side of the loop. This starts a current moving clockwise completely around the loop. The applicable equation is $F = qv \times B$. (Note: This method applies only if the loop is partially inside the field. If the loop were completely immersed in the field, the force on a charge on the opposite side of the loop would experience a force in the same direction, but the current direction would be in the opposite direction, so no net current would flow.)

A second approach to this problem is to apply Lenz's law. As the loop moves out of the magnetic field, the magnetic flux into the page decreases as more area of the loop moves out of the field. This decrease in flux into the page induces a current in the loop such that it creates a magnetic field to oppose the decrease. The current in the loop must be clockwise to create an increasing magnetic field *into* the page from the current in the loop to oppose the *decreasing* magnetic field into the page due to the decreasing flux. The direction of the induced current is determined by applying the "curled fingers" right-hand rule: curl your fingers in the direction of the current so that your extended thumb points into the page to represent the direction of the magnetic field from the induced current.

425. (D) The emf induced in the loop depends on the rate of change in flux.

$$\varepsilon = -\frac{\Delta\Phi}{\Delta t}$$

Since the loop makes 10 complete turns each second, one complete turn takes place in 0.1s. The flux, Φ, makes its maximum change when the wire turns one fourth of a cycle, that is, from a position where the loop is parallel to the field and there is no flux through the loop to a position where the loop is "open" to the field and flux is maximum. This quarter turn takes place in one fourth of 0.1 s. In this time, flux goes from 0 to its maximum, which is BA.

$$\Phi_{max} = BA = (80 \text{ T})(0.25 \text{ m}^2) = 20 \text{ Wb}$$

$$\varepsilon = \frac{\Delta\Phi}{\Delta t} = \frac{\Phi_f - \Phi_o}{\Delta t} = \frac{20 - 0}{(\frac{1}{4})(0.1)} = 800 \text{ V}$$

426. (D) When current is turned on to the larger solenoid, a magnetic field is produced inside the larger solenoid. Since the smaller solenoid is inside this magnetic field, a current will be induced in the wire of the smaller solenoid—but only at the instant the switch is turned on. At that moment, there is a change in magnetic flux to induce an emf in the smaller solenoid.

$$\varepsilon = \frac{\Delta\Phi}{\Delta t}$$

This induced emf, produced by the change in flux from zero to whatever it is inside the larger solenoid, produces a current in the smaller solenoid that depends on the resistance of the smaller solenoid. However, the emf and current are induced only at the moment the switch is turned on; once the current is steady, there is no longer an emf induced in the smaller solenoid, because there is no change in magnetic flux.

427. (A) By connecting the larger solenoid to an alternating power supply, the current in the larger solenoid alternates, the magnetic field produced by the larger solenoid also changes, which produces a changing magnetic flux as long as the larger solenoid is connected to the AC source. The changing magnetic flux induces a continuing (but also alternating) current in the smaller solenoid as long as the larger solenoid is connected to the AC source.

Chapter 13: Light and Optics

428. (C) Since $c = f\lambda$, where the speed of light, c, is constant, the frequency must be inversely proportional to wavelength. All of the other statements are true: all forms of electromagnetic radiation travel at the same speed (c) in a vacuum, all can be polarized, and all are formed of mutually perpendicular oscillating electric and magnetic fields.

429. (B) The lowest frequency forms of electromagnetic radiation have the longest wavelength and the lowest energy—which starts at the radio wave end of the spectrum. Here is a list of 11 types of electromagnetic radiation, in order from lowest frequency and longest wavelength to highest frequency and shortest wavelength: radio, infrared, red, orange, yellow, green, blue, violet, ultraviolet, X-ray, gamma. Choice (B)'s list is therefore in the correct order. Note that within the visible range of electromagnetic radiation, the color red has the longest wavelength, lowest frequency, and lowest energy. The visible colors, in order from longest wavelength to shortest wavelength, are identified by the acronym R-O-Y-G-B-V ("Roy G. Biv" without the indigo, which is not considered a distinct color).

430. (B) Visible light falls within a range of about 400 nm (at the violet end of the visible range) to 750 nm (at the red end of the visible range). Since ultraviolet light has a higher frequency and shorter wavelength than violet, ultraviolet light is in the range shorter than is visible to us: the 250–300 nm range. Choice (A) falls within the visible range—green to yellow. Choice (C) falls within the visible range—green to blue. Choice (D) falls within the red visible range. Light wavelengths longer than about 750 nm are in the infrared range, and not visible.

431. (D) Diffraction of light is evidence of the wave nature of light. Light has a dual nature—as photons that behave as particles and as waves that can interfere constructively when they are in phase and destructively when they are out of phase (for example, the crest of the wave pattern from one slit superimposed on the trough of the wave pattern from the second slit). The other choices are nonsense. In choice (A), light does have a particle nature and photons do have momentum, but they can't cancel when they collide, because energy would not be conserved. In choice (B), light is attenuated, or absorbed, by the region around the slits, but the remaining light would still create an interference pattern. In choice (C), it is the wave nature of light that causes diffraction of wave fronts as they pass through the slits, and those diffraction patterns interfere to produce a pattern.

432. (A) Geometrically, the distance from each slit to the center of the diffraction pattern is the same, so the path length difference is zero. Since there is only one monochromatic light source, it can be assumed that the waves pass through the slits in the same phase. Since they travel the same distance to the center of the pattern and start in the same phase, they will be in the same phase to produce constructive interference at the center of the pattern, which is called the "central maximum."

433. (C) Green light will change phase on its first reflection from the upper surface of the film, since the film has a higher index of refraction than air. In addition, green light will change phase after it goes into the film and reflects from the interface between the film and the glass. Since both reflections change phase, they will be in phase with each other and constructively interfere with each other as they reflect back out into air, *as long as* the trip of the light for the second reflection does not change the phase. Therefore, the trip down into the film and back out to air (which is twice the thickness of the film) must be an integral number of wavelengths of the green light *in the film*. If $2d = \lambda$, then $d = \lambda/2$.

434. (A) The numerous colors seen on a soap bubble result from the interference of reflected light from the top surface of the film with reflected light from the bottom surface of the film. The film has various thicknesses, so the colors are a result of constructive interference of the reflected light rays from the two surfaces of the film.

435. (A) Diffraction is the bending of waves as they pass through an opening or around an obstacle. Diffusion, which is not one of the choices, is the scattering of waves as they interfere with a medium. Reflection is a reversal in path as a wave strikes a boundary between two different media. Refraction is a change in path and wave speed as a wave moves from one medium into another. Dispersion is the separation of white light into component colors due to differences in refractive index for different colors.

436. (C) When applying the equation to a single slit, the integer designated by m applies to the dark fringes. When applying the same equation to a double slit, the integer applies to the bright fringes.

437. (B) The equation $m\lambda = d \sin \theta$ is used, where m is the number of the dark fringe, λ is the wavelength of the light, d is the aperture width, and θ is the angle for fringe spacing. As wavelength is increased (on one side of the equation), d is assumed to stay the same, and as a result, increases (on the other side of the equation). This will spread out the pattern of bright and dark fringes.

438. (A) The equation $m\lambda = d \sin \theta$ is used, where m is the number of the bright interference pattern from the central maximum, λ is the wavelength of the light, d is the spacing between lines on the grating, and θ is the angle swept by the bright lines from the central maximum to the bright line designated by m. If other conditions remain the same, changing to green light substitutes a smaller wavelength. Therefore, the angle θ would also become smaller, which results in a compression of the pattern on the screen.

439. (A) When the angles are very small (as in the case where d is proportionally large), the approximation in choice (A) is acceptable. For very small angles (measured in radians), the angle measurement is very close to the sine of the angle. This small angle approximation can be used in such cases, where $\theta = \dfrac{m\lambda}{d}$.

440. (D) Electromagnetic radiation is polarized as the electric field component of the radiation is affected by some materials. Choices (A), (B), and (C) are all examples of electromagnetic waves. Sound waves are longitudinal waves that travel only through a medium, are not electromagnetic, and cannot be polarized as they travel through a fluid (such as a gas or liquid). The direction of travel and direction of oscillation are the same—not perpendicular, as in electromagnetic oscillations.

441. (C) The intensity of light is reduced by half as it passes through a polarizer, because the electric field portion of the light is cut out, leaving only the magnetic field to contribute to the energy of the light.

442. (C) When the beam reflected from a surface is perpendicular to the refracted beam, the reflected beam is completely polarized in a direction parallel to the reflecting surface. This occurs when the incident angle is a special angle called "Brewster's angle," under the condition that the incident angle (Brewster's angle) plus the refracted angle must be 90 degrees. Polarization of light by reflection occurs on nonmetallic surfaces.

443. (B) As a distant object, such as a quasar, moves away from Earth, light from the object undergoes a "red shift," which is a decrease in frequency or increase in wavelength, which makes the light from the object shift toward the red end of the visible spectrum. This is true for any radiation coming from the distant object—observed radiation that is of longer wavelength than at the source.

444. (B) Total internal reflection occurs when light from a material with a higher index of refraction crosses an interface to a material with a lower index of refraction. In this situation, the light refracts away from the normal in the second medium, while some light reflects back into the original medium. As the incident angle is increased in size, the refracted angle also increases, and more of the light is also reflected back into the medium. When the incident angle is the critical angle, the refracted angle is 90°. Beyond that point, as the incident angle increases beyond the critical angle, all of the light is reflected back into the original medium.

445. (B) The image of a person standing in front of a plane (uncurved) mirror appears to that person to be "flipped" horizontally but not vertically, so it appears to be an upright image. Since the light rays don't actually pass through the point where the image appears (behind the mirror), the image is virtual. Since the image appears to be the same distance behind the mirror as the person is standing in front of the mirror, the distance of the image behind the mirror is d, and the distance of the image from the person is $2d$.

446. (B) Ray B does not follow a valid path after reflection from the mirror. Ray C follows an incident path parallel to the principal axis, so it correctly reflects through the focal point. Ray A correctly follows an incident path through the focal point, so it correctly reflects parallel to the principal axis. Ray D follows an incident path to the center of the lens, so it reflects at an equal angle to the principal axis.

447. (B) The index of refraction, n, of a medium is defined as the ratio of the speed of light in a vacuum to the speed of light in the medium. A low index of refraction indicates that the speed of light in the medium is closer to the speed of light in a vacuum; a high index of refraction indicates a larger ratio of speed in a vacuum to speed in the medium. Thus, the higher the n value, the slower light travels. As light enters a medium of index of refraction n, its speed and wavelength are both reduced by the same ratio. The frequency of the light does not change when it is refracted.

448. (D) Convex mirrors and concave lenses both cause light rays to diverge, so neither can produce real images under any conditions. Concave mirrors and convex lenses can produce real images, but only if the object is placed outside the focal point. Plane mirrors do not focus light, so they produce only virtual images. In choice (D), a concave lens does not focus light, so it cannot produce a real image.

449. (D) The thin-lens equation is used with the quantities provided to find a value for f in terms of d_o. If the magnification is one half (that is, the image is half as tall as the object), the ratio of the image distance, d_i, to the object distance, d_o, is ½.

$$\frac{1}{f} = \frac{1}{d_o} + \frac{1}{d_i}$$

$$\frac{1}{-f} = \frac{1}{d_o} + \frac{1}{½d_o}$$

$$\frac{1}{-f} = 3d_o$$

$$d_o = -3f$$

$$-f = \frac{d_o}{3}$$

450. (B) White light is composed of all the colors of visible light. The frequency of light does not change as it goes from one medium into another, but the speed and wavelength of each color do change. Index of refraction varies with color (and frequency), so each color refracts at a different angle, separating the white light into colors. This separation will not occur if the white light enters the glass or exits along a normal, so a flat piece of glass will not disperse the colors. Thus, a prism is constructed as an angular piece so that the white light passes at least one interface at an angle to disperse the light. Shorter wavelengths are refracted at a larger angle than longer wavelengths.

451. (D) Total internal reflection can only occur at an interface where the light is traveling from a medium with a higher index of refraction to a medium with a lower index of refraction. Under this condition, the incident angle must be greater than the critical angle: $\theta_c = \sin^{-1}(n_2/n_1)$, $n_1 > n_2$.

452. (D) Rays passing from the object through the lens will be directed parallel to each other on the other side of the lens, so they will not converge to form an image. This is confirmed by applying the thin-lens equation.

$$\frac{1}{d_o} + \frac{1}{d_i} = \frac{1}{f}$$

$$\frac{1}{f} + \frac{1}{d_i} = \frac{1}{f}$$

There is no real value for the image distance.

453. (C) A diverging (concave) lens cannot create a real image. (The only two possibilities for real images are an object positioned outside the focal length of a convex lens or a concave mirror.) A negative focal length is substituted into the thin-lens equation, as follows.

$$\frac{1}{d_o} + \frac{1}{d_i} = \frac{1}{f}$$

$$\frac{1}{12} + \frac{1}{d_i} = \frac{1}{-6}$$

$$\frac{1}{d_i} = -\frac{1}{6} - \frac{1}{12} = -\frac{3}{12}$$

$$d_i = -4$$

The image is located 4 cm from the lens, on the same side of the lens as the object, and is a virtual image. All virtual images are upright.

454. (D) The thin-lens equation is used, with $d_o = 1.5f$.

$$\frac{1}{d_o} + \frac{1}{d_i} = \frac{1}{f}$$

$$\frac{1}{1.5f} + \frac{1}{d_i} = \frac{1}{f}$$

$$\frac{2}{3f} + \frac{1}{d_i} = \frac{1}{f}$$

$$d_i = 3f$$

The positive image distance means the image is real, so it forms on the opposite side of the lens from the object.

455. (B) The index of refraction, n, is the ratio of the speed of the electromagnetic radiation in a vacuum to the speed of the radiation in the medium: $n = c/v$. Choice (B) is correct, because if $n = 1.5$, or 3/2, then the ratio c/v equals 3/2 and the ratio $v/c = 2/3$. Choice (A) is not correct, because frequency remains constant. Choice (C) is not correct, because a ray of light entering a medium along a perpendicular line (or normal line) changes speed and wavelength but does not change direction. Choice (D) is not correct, because it implies that light entering the medium travels at a speed faster than the speed of light.

456. (C) The thin-lens equation is used, and a negative value is used for the focal length.

$$\frac{1}{d_o} + \frac{1}{d_i} = \frac{1}{f}$$

$$\frac{1}{1.5f} + \frac{1}{d_i} = \frac{1}{-f}$$

$$\frac{2}{3f} + \frac{1}{d_i} = \frac{-1}{f}$$

$$d_i = -\frac{3f}{5}$$

The negative value for image distance indicates that the image forms on the same side of the lens as the object.

457. (B) We see only the colors reflected or transmitted to our eyes. If the object looks blue under a white light source, it reflects blue and absorbs all other visible colors, so the object is called blue. A yellow filter transmits only red and green light (since yellow is a composite of the primary colors of light—red and green). When the object is viewed through a yellow filter, the blue light reflected from the object is not transmitted by the yellow filter, so we see no colors transmitted from the object—and the object appears black.

458. (D) Each color of light has a different index of refraction in glass. Index of refraction relates the speed of light in a vacuum to the speed of light in a medium ($n = c/v$), with light of high frequency having a higher index of refraction. Frequency remains the same as each color travels into the glass, but both the speed and wavelength decrease, depending on the index. Thus, the blue end of the spectrum changes more—in speed, wavelength, and direction. The red end of the spectrum changes less. Choice (D) is correct, because blue light has a higher frequency than red and has a higher index—reducing speed more than red.

459. (C) Power in diopters is the reciprocal of focal length in meters. The first lens has power 1/0.5, or 2 diopters, and the second lens has power 1/0.25, or 4 diopters. Power in diopters is additive (this is the advantage of using diopters), so the power of the combination is 6 diopters.

460. (D) Lens strength in diopters is additive, so the strength of the combination is 3.25 diopters. The two lenses act as one lens with a focal length of 1/3.25. This fraction is quickly converted to 1/(13/4), or 4/13, which is closest to 0.33 m, or 33 cm.

461. (D) Aberration due to separation of colors (blue bending more than red toward a focal point) is called chromatic aberration.

462. (D) In nearsightedness, light from a distant source focuses at a "near" point after passing through the lens of the eye; the light is focused in front of the retina, making the image fuzzy to the person. A concave lens diverges the light, extending the focal point closer to the retina and helping the image to appear clear. People who are farsighted (hyperopic) use convex lenses to focus light on the retina when the light naturally focuses behind the retina (generally due to an eye structure that is "short" with respect to the shape of the lens or due to a lens that is unable to change shape to focus on the retina).

463. (C) The magnification of a microscope is determined by multiplying the magnifications of the eyepiece and objective lenses. In this case, the magnification is 50 times. The object on the slide is then seen as 50 times 0.3mm, or 15 mm. Since there are 10 mm per centimeter, the object appears to be 1.5 cm in diameter.

464. (C) Light from distant objects focuses from the objective lens at a point 15 cm from the lens, and then this serves as a real object for the eyepiece lens. If this image is at the focal point of the eyepiece lens, then the observer can view the image as if it were an infinity. The image, however, is now enlarged and can be viewed with a relaxed eye. Therefore, the sum of the focal lengths (15 cm + 5 cm) will be the length of the tube.

465. (A) Laser light may be polarized but is not necessarily so. However, laser light is monochromatic (in a single frequency) and coherent (with all waves in phase).

466. (C) For laser light to be produced, a metastable state must exist in which there is an inversion, that is, there are more electrons in the higher-energy metastable state than in a lower state. Photons with energy equal to the difference between the energy of the metastable state and a lower energy state pass near electrons in the metastable state, increasing the probability that they will emit photons that are of the same energy as the incident photons—and that are also in the same phase and moving in the same direction. The electrons then move to the lower energy state. Choice (A) is not correct, because the lower energy state is not necessarily the ground state and the emitted light is not necessarily visible. Choice (B) is not correct, because the photon energy is the energy *difference* between the metastable state and the lower energy state, which is not necessarily the ground state. Choice (D) is not correct, because photons are given off during the process and the metastable state is of higher energy than the ground state.

Chapter 14: Atomic and Nuclear Physics

467. (C) Since the energy of an emitted photon is being considered, only the transitions in choices (A) and (C) qualify. The transitions in choices (B) and (D) are absorptions, since they represent transitions from lower energy states to higher energy states. The highest frequency photon would be emitted for the transition of highest energy ($E = hf$). The energy emitted, ΔE, is equal to final energy minus original energy. Inspection of the diagram shows that the change in energy from $n = 3$ to $n = 1$ is greater than that from $n = 4$ to $n = 2$.

468. (D) In the derivation of energy states for the Bohr model of the atom, the energy of the lowest energy state is represented by E, or $n = 1$. The higher energy states for the electron are numbered consecutively and have energies equal to E/n^2. For example, if the energy for the ground state is -13.6 electron volts (eV), then the energy for the next higher state ($n = 2$) must be equal to $-13.6/2^2$, or -3.4 eV.

469. (D) The energy states of the Bohr model of the hydrogen atom have the lowest energy state, or ground state, labeled $n = 1$. Each subsequent higher allowed energy state has energy proportional to the square of the level number. For example, the next higher energy state from the ground state ($n = 2$) has one fourth the energy of the ground state, and the third energy state ($n = 3$) has one ninth the energy of the ground state. The average energy is also proportional to the inverse square of the distance from the nucleus, so the third energy state ($n = 3$) has one ninth the energy of the ground state and the electron would be nine times farther, on average, from the nucleus.

470. (C) The Rutherford model, which was developed prior to the Bohr model, emphasized the structure of the nucleus. The Bohr model, proposed in 1915, improved on the Rutherford model by emphasizing that (1) electrons orbit at only discrete energies and distances from the nucleus; (2) the energy of each orbit is related to its size, with smaller orbits having lower energy; and (3) radiation is emitted or absorbed when electrons transition from one energy state, or orbital, to another. The Bohr model is inaccurate in many ways—and now considered obsolete—but it is useful as a tool to calculate quantum transitions of electrons between energy levels.

471. (A) For angular momentum to be conserved, an integral number of electron wavelengths must "fit" into the orbit. The circumference of the orbit is $2\pi R$, so—according to the Bohr model—only an integral number of wavelengths (nR) would fit into that orbit without the electron wavelengths undergoing destructive interference. For the next energy level ($n + 1$), the allowed orbital has a radius and electron energy that must agree with the condition $2\pi R_{new} = (n + 1)\lambda_{new}$.

472. (A) One approach to the problem is to substitute $E = hf$, the expression for energy (E) related to frequency (f) using Planck's constant (h). The expression in choice (A) becomes hc/hf, which reduces to c/f. In considering $\lambda = c/f$, the expression $c = f\lambda$ becomes apparent—a true statement. Cross-multiplying the other choices produces nothing reasonable. For example, in choice (D), hf in the numerator is equal to E; the result is $\lambda = E/E = 1$, which is not a reasonable solution.

Considering the correct expression in choice (A), it becomes apparent that as the energy level increases, the wavelength must decrease (since h and c are constants). This makes sense: electrons in higher energy states do not have higher energy—they have higher frequency ($E = hf$), and higher frequency waves have longer wavelengths.

473. (D) Only the energy transitions shown are allowed. The arrows are the possible energy state transitions for absorbed photons—and their reverse in each case would be an emitted photon. The energy for each emission is $\Delta E = E_{final} - E_{initial}$. The smallest change possible is from the $n = 4$ state to the $n = 3$ state.

$$\Delta E = E_{final} - E_{initial} = -1.51 - (-0.85) = -0.66 \text{ eV}$$

The negative value on this change means that the energy is emitted in the form of a photon of this energy. The frequency of this photon could be calculated using the equation $E = hf$, where h is Planck's constant.

474. (C) The diagram is constructed so that the spacing indicates the amount of energy between the energy states. The transition from $n = 4$ to $n = 1$ is an allowed energy transition, and this transition would give off energy ($\Delta E = E_{final} - E_{initial} = -13.6 - (-0.85) = -12.75$ eV). The energy is directly proportional to frequency and inversely proportional to wavelength. Thus, this high energy transition would emit a photon with high energy and short wavelength.

475. (B) Change in energy state, ΔE, is equal to the energy of the final state minus the energy of the original state. If the transition is from higher energy to lower energy, the energy change is negative, which means that energy is given off in the form of light; that is the case here. If the final energy state is higher than the original energy state, the net change is positive, which means that energy is absorbed as photons of light. In the equation, h is Planck's constant. The substitution is based on the equation $c = f\lambda$, where c is the speed of light.

$$\Delta E = hf = \frac{hc}{\lambda}$$

$$\lambda = \frac{hc}{E_2 - E_1}$$

476. (D) The photoelectric effect is an example of conservation of energy. The energy of light photon absorbed (hf) is equal to the work necessary to strip each electron (called the work function, Φ) plus leftover energy used to give the electron kinetic energy.

$$hf = \Phi + K$$

The point at which the line intercepts the x axis is the lowest possible frequency that can result in electron emission; it is called the cutoff frequency, or threshold frequency. This frequency will supply enough energy to free the electron. This value is closest to 1×10^{15} Hz.

477. (C) This notation shows the composition of the nucleus of the atom. The lower number (on the left) is the atomic number, which is the number of protons in the nucleus; this identifies the element. The upper number is the mass number, which is the number of nucleons, or number of protons and neutrons in the nucleus. In a neutral atom, the number of electrons in the atom is equal to the number of protons in the nucleus.

478. (D) Protons and neutrons, which make up atomic nuclei, are called nucleons, so choice (A) is true. Since atomic nuclei increase in radius as they increase in mass, the density of atomic nuclei remains approximately constant, so choice (B) is true. The number of protons in the nucleus identifies the element, so choice (C) is true. However, the nuclei of atoms of the same element may vary in the number of neutrons, so the total number of nucleons in nuclei of the same element may vary; therefore, choice (D) is not true.

479. (C) The proton and neutron are both nucleons, or particles found in the nucleus of the atom. Both are composed of quarks, so neither is a fundamental particle. Fundamental particles, such as the electron or neutrino, do not have internal structure, as far as we now know. A deuteron is a nucleus composed of a proton and a neutron held together by nuclear forces and is thus not a fundamental particle. Another name for deuteron is deuterium nucleus, that is, an isotope of hydrogen that has a mass number of 2 due to the presence of the neutron.

480. (D) Hydrogen has three isotopes, that is, forms of hydrogen that have one proton in the nucleus (which identifies it as hydrogen). The isotope deuterium has one proton and one neutron in the nucleus, and the isotope tritium has one proton and two neutrons in the nucleus. These are the three isotopes of hydrogen: protium (^1_1H), deuterium (^2_1H), and tritium (^3_1H).

481. (D) Choices (A), (B), and (C) are all possible transformations within the nucleus. In each case, the charge after the reaction is the same as the charge before it. In choice (D), however, the charge before the transformation would be positive, and the total charge afterward would be negative—which does not conserve charge.

482. (B) For smaller elements, the ratio of neutrons to protons in stable nuclei tends to be 1:1. However, as the nuclei become larger in elements with increasing atomic number, stable nuclei tend to have a slightly larger ratio of neutrons to protons—closer to 1.6:1.

483. (D) The weak nuclear force is generally defined as the fundamental force responsible for beta decay (radioactivity). The force that causes electrons to be attracted to the positively charged nucleus is the electromagnetic force. The force, or interaction, that causes nucleons to attract and thus holds the nucleus together is the strong nuclear force. The force that causes protons to repel other protons is the electromagnetic force.

484. (C) At short ranges, that is, within the nucleus, the strong nuclear force is considered to be the strongest. The gravitational force is by far the weakest.

485. (B) The emission of an alpha particle (^4_2He, a helium nucleus with 2 protons and 2 neutrons) results in a new nucleus that has 2 fewer protons and 2 fewer neutrons. The loss of 2 protons and 2 neutrons reduces the mass number by 4.

486. (B) A beta particle is a high-speed electron, which has an atomic number of −1 and a mass number of 0: $^0_{-1}e$. To conserve charge, the new nucleus must have a higher atomic number by +1 to balance the −1 charge of the emitted electron. To conserve mass, there is no change in the mass number for the new nucleus, since the emitted electron has a mass number of 0.

487. (C) Emission of only one gamma photon would defy conservation of linear momentum. When two photons are emitted, they have components of momentum in opposite directions that add to zero, so no "new" momentum is created in a particular direction.

488. (C) The half-life is a probability of decay, so if there is only one nucleus, either it will decay or it will not. Therefore, the probability is 50% that the nucleus will have decayed.

489. (C) A beta⁻, or high-energy electron, would be produced from a nuclear neutron decay that also produced a proton. This is the only choice that involves decay, or breakdown of larger particles into smaller particles. It is also the only choice that obeys conservation of charge, that is, the total charge before the decay equals the total charge after the decay. In choice (C), the neutron has no charge before the decay, and the proton and electron have positive and negative charges, respectively, which add to zero. Even though the proton and electron are quite different, with very different masses, their charges are opposite and equal.

490. (C) This half-life curve shows the probability of the amount of the original material that is radioactive after a given length of time. If the original 100 g sample is initially radioactive, the plot predicts that after one half-life, only 50 g of the sample would be radioactive. Interpolating from the graph, the curve is at 50 g somewhere between 150 and 200 days.

491. (A) Positrons are the antiparticles of electrons; they have the same mass as electrons, but each positron has a positive charge. Positrons may be given off during radioactive decay of the nucleus. Beta particles, which are electrons, may be given off during the process of radioactive decay. Alpha particles, which are helium nuclei consisting of 2 protons and 2 neutrons, are also radioactive decay products. However, gamma rays are not particles with mass, even though they are given off during radioactive decay. Gamma photons have energy, but they do not qualify as particles with mass.

492. (B) Starting with the atomic number of bismuth (83), the emission of an alpha particle ($^4_2$He) reduces this number by 2, resulting in an atomic number of 81. The emission of an electron ($^{\ 0}_{-1}e$) increases the atomic number by one, bringing it to 82—or choice (B). It is possible to check this answer by determining the mass number changes. Starting with a mass number of 215, giving off an alpha particle would reduce the mass number by 4, leaving the product with a mass number of 211. Giving off an electron does not change the mass number, so the final mass number remains 211—or choice (B).

493. (C) Alpha particles and positrons, which are positively charged, and beta particles, which are negatively charged, would all have a magnetic force exerted on them by the magnetic field, causing them to change direction: $F_B = qv \times B$. Gamma rays do not carry a charge, so they would pass undeflected through the magnetic field.

494. (D) The atomic charge (the bottom numbers) on both sides of the equation must balance due to conservation of charge, and the atomic mass (the top numbers) on both sides must balance due to conservation of mass. The total atomic charge (92) is already the same on both sides, so the missing product cannot have a charge. This fact eliminates choices (A), (B), and (C), since all of these have charges. The total atomic mass on the left is 236 and the total mass on the right is 233, so a mass of 3 is needed to balance the equation. Three neutrons would have this mass, as can be seen from the neutron on the left side of the equation.

495. (C) The atomic charge (the bottom numbers) on both sides of the equation must balance due to conservation of charge, and the atomic mass (the top numbers) on both sides must balance due to conservation of mass. The total atomic charge on the left is 4 and the total atomic charge on the right is 2, so two more positive charges are needed on the right side to balance the equation. Thus, choice (D) is eliminated. The total atomic mass on the left is 4 and the total mass on the right is 4, so the missing product must have zero mass. Positrons have zero mass, whereas a helium nucleus and protons both have mass.

496. (B) The atomic charge (the bottom numbers) on both sides of the equation must balance. Since the total is 2 on both sides, the unknown particle must have zero charge. Of the four choices, only a neutron has zero charge; this eliminates choices (A), (C), and (D). This can be checked by balancing the nucleon number, or mass number, on both sides; these are the top numbers. The total mass number on the left is 5 and the total mass number on the right is 4, so the unknown particle must have a mass number of 1. Only the neutron has no charge and a mass number of 1.

497. (A) The equation for momentum of a particle is $p = mv$. All of a photon's mass is in the form of energy, $E = mc^2$. In addition, the speed of the photon is the speed of light, c. Recognizing that the energy of a photon is $E = hf$, these values are substituted into the momentum equation.

$$p = mv = \left(\frac{E}{c^2}\right)(c) = \frac{E}{c} = \frac{hf}{c}$$

498. (B) MeV/c^2 is a convenient unit to use for the mass of a subatomic particle. From the equation $E = mc^2$, mass could be represented as any energy unit divided by c^2 (the speed of light squared). The electron volt (eV) is a unit of energy, defined as the amount of energy needed to move one electron through a potential difference of one volt, or 1.6×10^{-19} J. The MeV is a "mega electron volt," or 1,000,000 eV.

499. (B) When a nucleus in an excited state emits a gamma photon, the nucleus is left in a state of lower energy, but with no change in mass number, atomic number, or number of nucleons. The nucleus, however, has less mass, corresponding to the energy of the gamma photon. This reduction in mass can be calculated using $E = mc^2$.

500. (C) The mass of each particle is converted to energy, using the equation $E = mc^2$. Antiparticles have the same mass, so the total energy converted from the mass of the two particles is $2mc^2$. This energy is the energy of the two gamma photons that are produced, each of the same energy. The energy of a photon is $E = hf$, where h is Planck's constant and f is the frequency of the photon. Since there are two photons produced in the annihilation of the particle-antiparticle pair, the total energy of the photons is $2hf$, where f is the frequency of each photon. The two expressions are set equal to each other, and the equation is solved for f.

$$2hf = 2mc^2$$

$$f = \frac{mc^2}{h}$$